PUBLIC HEALTH IN THE 21ST CENTURY

LEAD EXPOSURE AND POISONING

CLINICAL SYMPTOMS, MEDICAL MANAGEMENT AND PREVENTIVE STRATEGIES

PUBLIC HEALTH IN THE 21ST CENTURY

Additional books in this series can be found on Nova's website under the Series tab.

Additional e-books in this series can be found on Nova's website under the e-book tab.

PUBLIC HEALTH IN THE 21ST CENTURY

LEAD EXPOSURE AND POISONING

CLINICAL SYMPTOMS, MEDICAL MANAGEMENT AND PREVENTIVE STRATEGIES

LEONARD HORTON
EDITOR

NOVA BIOMEDICAL
New York

Library of Congress Cataloging-in-Publication Data

ISBN: 978-1-63482-699-0
Library of Congress Control Number: 2015937675

Published by Nova Science Publishers, Inc. † New York

Contents

Preface

Lead is a heavy metal used since ancient times and is still employed for several industrial purposes due to its suitable physical and chemical properties. It is non-biodegradable and is very persistent in the environment. Human exposure can lead, however, to a wide range of biological effects. Lead (Pb) exposure is known to induce a wide range of physiological and biochemical dysfunctions in humans and animals. This books reviews works collected in international literature dealing with the effects of lead; the environmental contamination of lead and its associated public health risks; the influence of lead at different doses on the structure of intestinal microbial community in vivo and its relationships to intestinal epithelium in vitro; and finally, the effects of fractions of the edible halophyte, Sarcocornia perennis on human kidney cells after Pb intoxication.

Chapter I – Lead is a heavy metal used since ancient times in domestic tools, ammunitions, ornaments, statuettes, pigments and cosmetics, and is still employed for several industrial purposes due to its suitable physical and chemical properties. Lead is non-biodegradable and is very persistent in the environment; despite the progressive reduction in its applications, it is a common environmental and occupational contaminant widely distributed around the world. Human exposure to lead can result in a wide range of biological effects. Toxicity of lead has been extensively studied; adverse health effects caused by this metal include neurotoxicity, nephrotoxicity, and deleterious effects on the hematological and cardiovascular systems. The International Agency for Research on Cancer classified lead as possible human carcinogen (group 2B) and inorganic lead compounds as probable human carcinogens (group 2A); nevertheless, there is still controversy regarding its mutagenic, clastogenic and carcinogenic properties. This chapter reviews works collected so far in the international literature dealing with effects of lead on the genetic material. Studies including different genotoxicity parameters and experimental designs (*in vitro*, *in vivo*, human epidemiological) are covered.

Chapter II – *Background:* High volume of automobiles imported into Nigeria are fairly used. Due to the resultant effect of the high rate of road accidents and ambient air temperature which cause expansion and contraction on these vehicles, they undergo wear and tear as could be seen by the caking and flaking of the paint coatings. The vehicles are then taken to the car painting workshops for reworking (scrapping and repainting). *Method:* About fifty-six (56) scrapped paint dusts from 56 vehicles were collected from eight (8) different car paint workshops in south eastern Nigerian. They were homogenized, mixed and divided into fine particles that can pass through 0.5mm sieve and digested by standard method. The filtrates were assayed with atomic absorption spectrophotometry (AAS 200A). *Results:* Show that the lead (Pb) concentration were in the range of (1.42 ± 0.01 - 4.16 ± 0.01mg/kg) for workshop 1, (0.49 ± 0.01-3.50 ± 0,01mg/kg) for workshop2, (2.45 ± 0.01-4.36 ± 0.04mg/kg) for workshop 3, (2.94 ± 0.02-4.17 ± 0.00mg/kg) for workshop 4, etc; Dose exposure and risk assessment through inhalation and dermal contact were below USA EPA threshold limit. *Conclusion:* Reworking (scrapping and repainting) of fairly used vehicles imported into Nigeria may contribute to environmental lead burden with its associated public health risks.

Chapter III – Soluble forms of lead Pb(II) are well known toxins, entering organisms of humans and animals predominantly orally. Intestinal microflora represents a necessary functional component of the body and, together with intestinal epithelium, is usually subjected to the highest Pb(II) concentrations. This implies the importance of detailed study of lead impact in this particular context. The aim of our study was to investigate the influence of lead at different doses on the structure of the intestinal microbial community *in vivo* (rat) and its relationships to intestinal epithelium *in vitro*. In our experiments, lead doses that were much lower than those causing visible harmful effects on cell culture or on the level of the whole body, induced significant changes in intestinal microflora. Oral exposure to Pb created selective advantages for lactose-negative coli-forms and thus contributed into dysbacteriosis development. We suppose that the lead-induced dysbacteriosis was initiated by the changes in bacterial adhesion to the intestinal epithelium. This might be related to increased intestinal epithelium permeability also caused by lead, as it was shown in another series of our studies shown here. Furthermore, model dynamic light scattering measurements have revealed strong aggregating effect of lead on protein (albumin) solutions. The results could be possibly extrapolated to human beings, opening the opportunity to understand some mysterious cases of persisting dysbacteriosis as a result of latent Pb-intoxication. This, in turn, suggests a probiotic treatment as a promising therapy for lead-exposed patients on one hand and possible success of Pb-scavenging therapy for some patients with dysbacteriosis on the other hand.

Chapter IV – Lead (Pb) exposure is known to induce a wide range of physiological and biochemical dysfunctions in humans and animals. We previously showed that lead causes oxidative damage and cytotoxicity in human kidney cells. Now, we report the effects of fractions of the edible halophyte *Sarcocornia perennis* on these cells after Pb intoxication. HEK 293 cells were seeded in 96-well plates in medium containing Pb with or without fractions of *S. perennis* methanolic extract. Morphological and biochemical indicators were used to evaluate cytoprotective and antioxidant effects of the extract fractions. Our results showed that lead induced (1) a decrease in cell viability, (2) apoptosis, (3) cell distortion and cohesion loss, and (4) superoxide anion production and lipid peroxidation. These observations were alleviated upon addition of $MeOH_{80}$ fraction of plant extract and, to a lower extent, $MeOH_{60}$ one. Our results suggest that *S. perennis* contains promisful substances to counteract the lead intoxication.

In: Lead Exposure and Poisoning
Editor: Leonard Horton
ISBN: 978-1-63482-699-0

Chapter I

Lead Exposure: Assessment of Effects on the Genetic Material

María Sánchez-Flores[1,2], Blanca Laffon[1,*], Julia García-Lestón[1,2], Josefina Méndez[2], Eduardo Pásaro[1] and Vanessa Valdiglesias[1]

[1]DICOMOSA Group, Department of Psychology, Area of Psychobiology, Universidade da Coruña, Edificio de Servicios Centrales de Investigación, A Coruña, Spain
[2]Department of Cell and Molecular Biology, Universidade da Coruña, Faculty of Sciences, A Coruña, Spain

Abstract

Lead is a heavy metal used since ancient times in domestic tools, ammunitions, ornaments, statuettes, pigments and cosmetics, and is still employed for several industrial purposes due to its suitable physical and chemical properties. Lead is non-biodegradable and is very persistent in the environment; despite the progressive reduction in its applications, it is a common environmental and occupational contaminant widely distributed around the world. Human exposure to lead can result in a wide range of biological effects. Toxicity of lead has been extensively studied;

* E-mail: blaffon@udc.es

adverse health effects caused by this metal include neurotoxicity, nephrotoxicity, and deleterious effects on the hematological and cardiovascular systems. The International Agency for Research on Cancer classified lead as possible human carcinogen (group 2B) and inorganic lead compounds as probable human carcinogens (group 2A); nevertheless, there is still controversy regarding its mutagenic, clastogenic and carcinogenic properties. This chapter reviews works collected so far in the international literature dealing with effects of lead on the genetic material. Studies including different genotoxicity parameters and experimental designs (*in vitro*, *in vivo*, human epidemiological) are covered.

1. Introduction

Since ancient times, lead has been employed by human beings to make domestic tools, ammunitions, ornaments and statuettes. This is due to lead has unique physical and chemical properties, such as softness, malleability, ductility, poor conductibility and resistance to corrosion, along with its wide distribution on nature. The Romans were the first to use lead on a large scale in the manufacture of pipes for water supply, manufacture of tableware and kitchen utensils or even as additive to cosmetics and pigments, due to the bright characteristic colors of most lead compounds (black, white, yellow and red) (Delile et al., 2014; Hernberg, 2000; Robles-Osorio and Sabath, 2014; Thornton et al., 2001). Lead acetate was used later as a sweetener for wine and cider as well as in medicine for treating several diseases. The Industrial Revolution brought a dramatic increase in the use of lead worldwide and, later on, in the 1930s, discovery of antiknock and octane level strengthener properties of organic compound tetra-ethyl lead addition to gasoline largely contributed to its wide use and environmental dissemination (Thornton et al., 2001; Wedeen, 2011).

Lead poisoning was especially noticeable during the 16th to 19th centuries when its use was highly widespread whereas its toxic effects on human health had not been studied yet. Nowadays, exposure to lead has diminished due to the reduction of lead uses, but it is still present in many industrial activities, such as car repair, manufacturing and recycling of batteries, lead paint removal, demolition, refining and smeltery. It is also used for maintenance of structures found in the open air as bridges or water towers, in solders of cans of food or beverages, glazed ceramic, and can also be present in drinking water or in tobacco smoke (Patrick, 2006; Spivey, 2007). Environmental pollution caused by lead is persistent, due to the fact that it is a non-biodegradable element, and is extensively spread since lead has been widely used, and still is, in many products, affecting to population in general.

Lead toxicity is well known in several biological systems and functions. This toxicity was first described in childhood in early 20th century in the United States. A wider knowledge about lead toxicity effects in children was reached in 1940s when behavioral disorders and learning difficulties were related to lead poisoning. Then, lead-related deficits in intelligence quotient scores, attention and language were first reported in children in 1970s (Needleman, 2004). In this decade, also the first studies on lead effects were performed in adults, showing that peripheral and central nervous system, kidneys, and blood pressure were affected (Needleman, 2004; Wedeen, 2011).

In general, molecular processes of lead toxicity can be divided into three types (Minozzo et al., 2004): through binding to different electron donors, in particular sulfhydryl groups, changing protein conformation and enzymatic function through lead biochemical and biophysical similarity to essential polyvalent cations, and by affecting nucleic acids, what it is believed to be due to the production of free radicals.

Lead has the ability to inhibit essential cellular functions and to reach certain organs and organelles on which it exerts its effects, reason why lead can affect virtually all systems in the body (Silbergeld et al., 2000). Previous data point to the interferences with different enzymatic systems as the cause of this ability of inhibition through interaction with proteins. Lead can interfere by binding to sulfhydryl groups of the proteins or replacing essential divalent cations in different molecular processes (Silbergeld et al., 2000).

Nevertheless, lead genotoxic and carcinogenic properties are still controversial. The International Agency for Research on Cancer (IARC) classified lead as possible human carcinogen (group 2B) (IARC, 1987) and inorganic lead compounds as probable human carcinogens (group 2A) (IARC, 2006) on the basis of sufficient evidence for carcinogenicity in experimental animals but inadequate evidence for carcinogenicity in humans. Organic lead compounds cannot be classified as carcinogenic for humans (group 3) (IARC, 2006). Nevertheless, some epidemiological studies link exposure to lead to an elevated risk of stomach and lung cancers, and also of bladder and brain cancers (Fu and Boffeta, 1995; Rajaraman et al., 2006). However, later studies showed inconsistent results for bladder and brain/nervous system tumors, as well for kidney cancer (Gwini et al., 2012; Wilhelm et al., 2010). More recently, an increased cancer risk in both children (Cao et al., 2015) and adults

(Soltani et al., 2015) populations environmentally exposed to lead after dermal, digestive or inhalatory exposure pathways was confirmed.

To better understand the carcinogenetic properties of lead, several mechanism have been proposed, such as mitogenesis, alterations in gene transcription, oxidative damage and several indirect genotoxicity mechanisms (Hartwig, 1994; Silbergeld, 2003). However, it has been also suggested that lead plays an indirect role in carcinogenesis, increasing the risk of cancer by reducing the ability of cells to protect or repair DNA damaged by other exposures, rather than being the direct responsible of alterations in DNA (Kašuba et al., 2010; Silbergeld et al., 2000).

2. Studies of Lead Effects on Genetic Material

During cell division, the coordination of DNA replication with DNA-damage sensing and repair and cell-cycle progression is vital to ensure genome integrity, and prevent mutations and DNA rearrangements than can be harmful for the organism (Aguilera and Gómez-González, 2008). However, cellular genomes are constantly subjected to a variety of physical and chemical agents with the ability to produce mutations in essential genes of somatic cells, which can lead to potentially harmful diseases (Erickson, 2003; Li et al., 2014). The mutational events that may occur include point mutations, deletions, duplications, translocations, mitotic recombination, gene conversion, gene amplification and aneuploidy. As many of these mutational mechanisms are involved in the development of specific types of tumors in humans, measures of the frequency of different types of mutagenic events in human cells, both *in vivo* and *in vitro,* facilitate the study of the health risks associated with these events (Li et al., 2014; Loi et al., 2013; Olsen et al., 1996). For this purpose, several tests have been developed to determine the mutation frequency caused by mutagenic agents in somatic cells. Among them, the most frequently used are hypoxanthine-guanine phosphoribosyl-transferase (*hprt*) and T cell receptor (TCR) mutation assays.

Together with these assays, lead genotoxic effects have been traditionally evaluated by cytogenetic tests, which assess different types of structural and numeric chromosome alterations. The most representative ones are sister chromatid exchanges (SCE), micronucleus (MN) test, and chromosome aberrations (CA). However, among all the lesions that toxic compounds may cause in the genetic material of the exposed organisms, the most frequent and possibly the easiest to detect are breaks in the DNA strands (Bernstein and Bernstein, 1991). Many assays have been developed to evaluate these DNA alterations, such as the alkaline sucrose sedimentation (Humphrey et al., 1968; McBurney et al., 1972; Veatch and Okada, 1969), the alkaline unwinding (Rydberg, 1975; Taningher et al., 1987), or the alkaline elution (Bihari et al., 1990; Bolognesi et al., 1992, 1996; Kohn et al., 1976; Vukmirovic et al., 1994); but since almost three decades ago, the single cell gel electrophoresis (comet) assay has being more and more used due to its sensitivity and simplicity (Olive et al., 1990, 1991; Singh et al., 1988; Steinert et al., 1998; Wilson et al., 1998).

In order to evaluate genotoxicity associated with lead exposure, all these techniques can be applied on cell culture systems (*in vitro*), on experimental animals or whole organisms (*in vivo*) and on human populations (epidemiological studies). The following sections summarize studies describing the main effects of lead exposure on the genetic material published so far.

2.1. *In vitro* Studies

Mutagenicity

The mutagenic potential of lead has been usually evaluated *in vitro* by means of the *hprt* mutation assay. HPRT is a non-essential enzyme that phosphoribosylates free guanine or hypoxanthine for the synthesis of nucleic acids. In normal cells, HPRT catalyzes the conversion of the base analogue 6-thioguanine (TG) into a cytotoxic compound. This compound is introduced in the DNA and paralyzes replication resulting in cell death. Inactivating mutations of the *hprt* gene allow the mutant cells to grow in the presence of otherwise toxic concentrations of TG, providing a good medium for their selection by direct cloning (Albertini et al., 1993). The *hprt* gene is capable of reflecting a wide variety of genetic alterations such as DNA base pair substitutions, large and small deletions, inversions and heterologous chromosome recombinations (Albertini and Hayes, 1997; Cole and Skopek, 1994).

Most studies using this technique to evaluate the genotoxic effects of lead *in vitro* did not show any increase in the mutation frequency at the *hprt* locus (Hartwig et al., 1990; Hwua and Yang, 1998; Patierno et al., 1988; Patierno and Landolph, 1989). Only two studies (Yang et al., 1996; Zelikoff et al., 1988) found positive results.

Yang et al., (1996) evaluated the mutagenicity of lead acetate at the *hprt* gene of CHO K1 cells. Their results showed that lead acetate induced a dose-dependent mutant frequency at doses lower than the LD_{50}. To determine the mutational specificity induced by lead, cDNA and genomic DNA sequences were characterized. Sequencing analysis showed lead-induced single-base substitutions, small sequence alterations, splicing defects, and gene deletions. Although lead produced a broad mutational spectrum similar to that occurring spontaneously, the positions and kinds of base substitutions at the *hprt* gene induced by lead were different. The predominant mutations were G·C→C·G transversions in low-mutant-frequency populations and G·C→A·T transitions in high-mutant-frequency populations. These observations indicate that different lead mutagenic mechanisms may exist for inducing low and high mutant frequencies. On the contrary, Hwua and Yang (1998) did not find any increase in the mutation frequency at the *hprt* gene in diploid human skin fibroblasts (HFW) at similar cytotoxic dosages of lead acetate than those used by Yang et al., (1996). The fact that lead mutagenicity was observed in CHO K1 cells, but not in human fibroblasts, may be attributable, according to the authors, to the different defense mechanisms against lead genotoxicity in HFW and CHO K1 cells. In fact, the basal metallothionein (the most important metal-binding protein) level is approximately 5 μg/mg protein in HFW (Lin et al., 1995), but undetectable in CHO K1, and the catalase level is ≈ 50-fold higher in HFW than in CHO K1 (Hwua and Yang, 1998; Lee and Ho, 1995; Yang et al., 1996). This comparison suggests that metal mutagenicity is positively correlated to the cellular oxidative stress, i.e. mutation may be induced in cells having limited antioxidant machinery (Hwua and Yang, 1998).

McNeill et al., (2007) did not observe any increase in *hprt* gene mutation frequencies in both CHO AA8 and hApe1-3 cells exposed to lead. However, when both cell lines were exposed to lead in combination with methylmethanesulphonate (MMS), *hprt* mutagenesis significantly increased. These results indicate that while lead is a poor mutagen by itself, it can act as an effective co-mutagen in the presence of a DNA-damaging agent such as MMS.

Chromosome Alterations

As mentioned above, three different types of cytogenetic assays are mainly used to determine chemically induced changes in the structure or number of chromosomes: SCE, CA and MN test. SCE involve breakage of both DNA strands of a chromosome, followed by an exchange of whole DNA duplexes between sister chromatids. SCE events cannot be considered by themselves as mutations because they do not produce any changes in the genetic information. However, it appears that the frequency of SCE increases when cells are exposed to known carcinogens and mutagens. The *in vitro* studies that evaluated alterations in SCE rates induced by lead report contradictory results. Increases in the frequency of SCE were found when evaluating the genotoxic effects of different lead salts. Douglas et al., (1980) evaluated the effect of lead chromate on CHO cells; Wulf (1980) tested lead sulphate in human lymphocytes; Sharma et al., (1985) and Poma et al., (2003) investigated the induction of SCE by lead acetate in pregnant mice and their fetuses and in human melanoma cells (B-Mel), respectively; and Lin et al., (1994) and Cai and Arenaz (1998) used lead nitrate in CHO cells. On the other hand, no effect of lead on the frequency of SCE was observed by Beek and Obe (1974) and Hartwig et al., (1990), who evaluated the genotoxic effect of lead acetate on human leukocytes and on Chinese hamster V79 cells, respectively, and by Zelikoff et al., (1988), who assessed the genotoxicity of lead sulphide and lead nitrate in V79 cells. Furthermore, Montaldi et al., (1985) analyzed SCE induction by several heavy metal salts, including lead, in CHO cells and they observed that lead sulphate increased SCE frequency whereas lead acetate did not.

The chromosome aberrations (CA) test detects changes in the structure of chromosomes, which are visible under the optical microscope. These changes result from breaks and rearrangements within a chromosome or between different chromosomes. Such reorganizations are produced mainly by substances that directly break the DNA strand (e.g., radiation) or distort the DNA double helix (e.g., intercalating agents). The mode of action of a genotoxic agent will determine the type of chromosomal structural alterations produced. The CA test has been employed in numerous studies to evaluate the genotoxic effects induced by lead or its derivatives. Regarding *in vitro* studies, treatment of human leukocytes with lead acetate showed clearly elevated frequencies of achromatic lesions, chromatid breaks and isochromatid breaks in 72 h cultures, but not in 48 h cultures (Beek and Obe, 1975). Deknut and Deminatti (1978) observed that the most common aberration induced by lead acetate in human lymphocyte cultures was the occurrence of chromosome fragments. Also, Pottier et al., (2013) found telomere instability, both short and dysfunctional telomeres, in human bladder cells exposed to lead. On the contrary, Schmid et al., (1972) and Gasiorek and Bauchinger (1981) did not observe effect of lead acetate on the frequency of CA in human lymphocytes. Bauchinger and Schmid (1972) obtained the same negative results for Chinese hamster cells. Also, Asakura et al., (2009) obtained negative results for Chinese hamster cells treated with lead (purity: 99.9%). Other studies with lead nitrate and lead glutamate were also negative (Cai and Arenaz, 1998; Lin et al., 1994; Shaik et al., 2006). However, consistently positive results were obtained with lead chromate (Douglas et al., 1980; Wise et al., 1992; Wise et al., 1994, Wise et al., 2003; Wise et al., 2004; Xie et al., 2005; Xu et al., 1992), which most of the authors related to the probable action of chromate. Conversely, Nestman and Zhang (2007) obtained negative results with lead chromate, which they associate with the use of insoluble forms of lead chromate, opposite to soluble forms used in the studies with positive results.

During cell division, chromosome breakage due to unrepaired or mis-repaired DNA lesions, and/or chromosome malsegregation due to mitotic malfunction, lead to formation of MN. These events may be induced by oxidative stress, exposure to clastogens or aneugens, genetic defects in cell cycle checkpoints and/or DNA repair genes, as well as deficiencies in nutrients required as co-factors in DNA metabolism and chromosome segregation machinery (Bonassi et al., 2007). MN can derive from acentric chromosome fragments or whole chromosomes that are left behind (lagging chromosomes) during anaphase movements (Carrano and Natajaran, 1988). MN containing chromosome fragments result from: (a) direct DNA breakage; (b) replication on a damaged DNA template; or (c) inhibition of DNA synthesis. While MN containing whole chromosomes are primarily formed from failure of the mitotic spindle, kinetochore, or other parts of the mitotic apparatus, or by damage to chromosomal sub-structures, alterations in cellular physiology, and mechanical disruption. Therefore, the MN frequency can be used as a biomarker of genotoxic effects that reflect exposure to agents with clastogenic or aneugenic modes of action. This assay presents some advantages in comparison to other cytogenetic genotoxicity tests (Albertini and Kirsch-Volders, 1997; Miller et al., 1997): potential of detecting clastogenic and aneugenic compounds; simplicity of the method; fast and inexpensive; higher statistical power (due to the fact that many cells are analyzed); potential for automation using image analysis; and possibility to obtain mechanistic information in combination with other techniques. However the assay has some disadvantages since it does not detect all the structural chromosomal aberrations, only acentric fragments, and it requires pre-division for the expression of MN.

Poma et al., (2003) found that lead acetate induced MN in a dose-dependent manner when evaluated chromosomal damage induced in human melanoma cells (B-Mel). Thier et al., (2003) and Bonacker et al., (2005) studied the genotoxic effects of inorganic lead salts in V79 Chinese hamster fibroblasts by means of MN test. They observed that lead chloride and lead acetate induced MN in a dose-dependent manner, and they determined by means of antikinetochore antibody staining that the effects of lead were predominantly aneugenic, which was consistent with the observed morphology of the MN. Moreover, Sandhu et al., (1989) assessed the clastogenic potential of various chemicals commonly found at industrial waste sites by means of MN test. They found positive results for lead in plant cuttings of Tradescantia clone 4430. To our knowledge, only one MN *in vitro* study showed negative results for lead so far (Lin et al., 1994). In this study the authors investigated the effects of cadmium nitrate and lead nitrate on CHO cells by means of a number of short-term assays, including the MN test. They found that lead nitrate did not significantly increase MN frequencies.

Primary DNA Damage

The technique most commonly used to evaluate the primary DNA damage is the single cell gel electrophoresis assay, also known as comet assay. It is a simple, rapid and sensitive method for the analysis and quantification of DNA damage, particularly DNA breaks, at the level of individual cells, which can be applied to practically all cell types and can thereby detect genotoxic effects induced by different physical or chemical agents. DNA damage detected by the alkaline version of the assay can arise through various mechanisms, including DNA double- and single-strand breaks, alkali-labile sites, DNA inter-strand cross-linking, and incompletely repaired excision sites present at the time of lysis. Compared with other genotoxicity tests, the advantages of this technique include (Olive and Banath, 2006; Rojas et al., 1999; Tice, 1995; Tice et al., 2000): (1) data are collected at the level of individual cells, providing information on the intercellular distribution of damage and repair, (2) only a small number of cells is required, (3) almost any eukaryotic cell population can be used, (4) the assay is sensitive, simple and cost effective, (5) data can be obtained within a few hours of sampling, (6) a relatively short time period (a few days) is needed to complete an experiment, (7) the assay can evaluate DNA damage in non-proliferating cells, (8) cells do not need to be tagged with a radioisotope, thus allowing measurement of damage in any nucleated cell; (9) the method could be used to measure variations in response to DNA damaging agents between cells of the same exposed population, and (10) it has a demonstrated sensitivity for detecting low levels of DNA damage.

Few studies were conducted *in vitro* to evaluate the genotoxicity of lead by means of the comet assay. In all of them a significant increase in DNA fragmentation was found when different cell types were exposed to lead salts. Robbiano et al., (1999) obtained significant dose-dependent increases of DNA strand breaks in primary rat and human kidney cells exposed to different concentrations of lead acetate. Wozniak and Blasiak (2003) evaluated the genotoxic effects of the same salt on human lymphocytes. They found an increase in the comet tail length due to the induction of DNA strand breaks and/or alkali labile sites. Lymphocytes exposed to the highest dose showed a decrease in the comet parameter caused by the formation of DNA-DNA and DNA-protein cross-links. In the same study, the neutral version of the assay revealed that lead acetate induced DNA double-strand breaks at all concentrations tested. Similarly, Shaik et al., (2006) found a significant increase in the comet tail length when they analyzed human lymphocytes exposed to lead nitrate, and this increase was proportional to lead nitrate concentration. Ahmad and Shakoori (2013) tested the genotoxic effect of lead nitrate in adipose derived mesenchymal stem cells. Fragmentation of DNA was observed in cells treated with lead nitrate after being stained with ethidium bromide. Monteiro et al., (2010) used *Prochilodus lineatus* erythrocytes to test lead nitrate genotoxicity by comet assay. Cells exposed to lead nitrate showed significant increases in the score of DNA damage in relation to controls. More recently, Sanders et al., (2014) studied the effect of lead nitrate on pheochromocytoma (PC-12) cell line, showing a concentration-dependent increase in DNA damage with chemical exposure; and Zhang et al., (2014) explored indirect DNA damage in mice liver cells induced by lead (Pb^{+2}), at different concentrations, by means of alkaline comet assay. Cells treated at all concentrations of lead showed increases in the comet parameters.

Supporting the comet assay results, a recently published study reported the emergence of γH2AX foci, commonly correlated with the formation of DNA double-strand breaks, some hours after exposure of human endothelial HMEC cells to lead (Gastaldo et al., 2007).

Effects on DNA Repair

DNA damage may be due to direct genotoxic insults or the consequence of alterations induced on the DNA repair mechanisms. Hartwig et al., (1990) investigated whether the genotoxicity of lead could be due to indirect effects, such as interference with DNA repair processes, by means of SCE among other endpoints. They found that lead acetate alone did not induce SCE in V79 Chinese hamster cells. However, lead ions enhanced the number of UV-induced SCE, suggesting that lead interfered with the processing of UV-induced DNA lesions. The authors reached the conclusion that not only the DNA damage itself but also the genotoxic effects of other chemical or physical agents may be augmented when repair is inhibited, as illustrated by the enhancement of UV-induced SCE.

Another study reported that lead nitrate contamination inhibited non-homologous end-joining DNA repair process by preventing the DNA protein kinase activity. This generated late unrepairable double-strand breaks that impact upon the ATM-dependent stress signaling pathway by favoring propagation of errors (Gastaldo et al., 2007). More recently, Gadhia et al., (2012) treated mouse embryonic stem cells with different trace elements, including lead, and observed that this compound reduced significantly the expression levels of relevant genes, namely *Rad-18*, *Top-3α* and *Ogg-1*, associated with DNA repair mechanisms.

2.2. *In vivo* Studies

Mammalian Studies

Only four studies conducted in animals evaluated the influence of lead on the frequency of SCE. Willems et al., (1982) investigated the effect of lead on SCE rate in male rabbits after exposure to different doses of lead acetate subcutaneously injected three times a week during 14 weeks. Statistical analysis of the number of SCE per metaphase in lymphocytes indicated no differences among groups. Nayak et al., (1989) analyzed the frequency of SCE in maternal bone marrow and fetal liver and lung cells of ICR Swiss Webster mice, following maternal exposure to lead nitrate. Lead caused a moderate, but statistically significant, increase in the frequency of SCE in maternal bone marrow cells. On the contrary, lead did not cause any effect on the frequency of SCE in liver or lung cells of fetus, although lead was shown to cross the placenta. Dhir et al., (1993) reported that intraperitoneal injection of low doses of lead nitrate caused a significant increase in SCE rate in bone marrow of male Swiss albino mice. Tapisso et al., (2009) studied the effect of lead acetate on bone marrow cells of male Algerian mice exposed to different number of doses (5 or 10). They observed a significantly increase in the frequency of SCE in all treated animals with regard to the controls, and higher SCE frequencies in those that received 10 doses.

CA assay was performed in a number of mammalian studies: leukocytes from male and female mice fed with lead acetate (Muro and Goyer, 1969), in lymphocytes from cynomolgus monkeys (*Macaca irus*) administered lead acetate in the diet (Jacquet and Tachon, 1981), in bone marrow cells of mice exposed daily to lead acetate (Huang et al., 1985), in bone marrow cells of rats after intraperitoneal administration of lead acetate (Tachi et al., 1985), in maternal bone marrow and fetal liver and lung cells of ICR Swiss Webster mice following maternal exposure to lead nitrate (Nayak et al., 1989), and in bone marrow cells from Swiss albino male mice orally gavaged to leachates (Tewari et al., 2005). All these studies showed significant increases in CA rates.

Other studies reported differential induction of several types of CA. Jacquet et al., (1977) carried out an experiment in which dietary lead acetate at different dose levels was given to female C57B1 mice for periods up to three months. They found no severe chromosome or chromatid aberrations at any dose level, but the frequency of chromatid gaps increased significantly at the highest doses. Deknudt et al., (1977a) described that the type of CA induced by lead acetate in cynomolgus monkeys (*Macaca irus*) depended on the intake of calcium in the diet. The frequency of severe abnormalities (dicentrics, rings, translocations and exchanges) was significantly increased only in the group on a low calcium diet, whereas "light" abnormalities (gaps and fragments) increased with time in all groups receiving lead irrespective of the diet. Aboul-Ela (2002) found only structural aberrations, like chromatid gaps, deletions and fragments, in bone marrow cells of male Swiss mice after oral administration of lead acetate. Nehéz et al., (2000) investigated the possible genotoxic effects exerted by the pyrethroid insecticide cypermethrin and by either of the metals cadmium and lead alone or in combination, on bone marrow cells of outbred male Wistar rats. Treatment with lead acetate only increased significantly the number of aberrant cells and numerical aberrations but did not alter the number of structural aberrations. The combination of cypermethrin and lead caused a significant increase in aberrant cells and in structural aberrations but not in numerical aberrations. The most frequently structural aberrations observed were gaps and acentric fragments. These results agree with Lorencz et al., (1996) who found increases in numerical aberrations in bone marrow cells from Wistar rats treated with different doses of lead acetate.

Also, several studies evaluated the genotoxic effects of lead acetate in rats by means of the MN test (Celik et al., 2005; Piao et al., 2007; Tachi et al., 1985; Tapiso et al., 2009). Most of them found an increase in the frequency of

MN after lead exposure. For instance, Alghazal et al., (2008) analyzed the MN rate in bone marrow erythrocytes of Wistar rats treated with lead acetate trihydrate and found a significant increase in the total number of MN in polychromatic erythrocytes of both male and female rats with regard to the control group. Similarly, Jagetia and Aruna (1998) observed an increase in the frequency of MN in bone marrow cells of mice treated with lead nitrate. The frequency of MN did not show a dose related increase, but male mice were more sensitive to the induction of MN than female mice, evidenced by higher frequencies of micronucleated polychromatic erythrocytes. In another work, Tewari et al., (2005) investigated the genotoxic potential of a leachate, a mixture of various organic chemicals and heavy metals among which lead is included, prepared from municipal sludge sample, in mouse bone marrow cells by MN test. Male mice orally gavaged to leachates revealed also a significant increase in micronucleated polychromatic erythrocytes. In this case, the cause of genotoxic effects may be due to one component or to combination of toxicants in the leachate. And more recently, lead was reported to induce increases in MN and SCE frequencies, together with sperm abnormalities, in mice treated intraperitoneally (Tapisso et al., 2009). Opposite to all these works, two studies carried out in mice (Jacquet et al., 1977) and rabbits (Willems et al., 1982) did not find any increase in the MN frequency in the group of animals exposed to lead acetate.

All studies conducted in animals using the comet assay showed a positive effect of lead on the induction of DNA damage in several tissues and organs. Valverde et al., (2002) used a lead acetate inhalation model in mice in order to detect the induction of genotoxic damage like single-strand breaks and alkali-labile sites in several organs. They found a positive induction of DNA damage after a single inhalation only in the liver and the lung. In subsequent inhalations the response was positive in all organs tested except for the testicle. These results showed that lead acetate inhalations induced systemic DNA damage but some organs are special targets for this metal, such as lung and liver, depending in part on length of exposure. Devi et al., (2000) also found a significant increase in mean comet tail length at any time intervals (24, 48, 72 h, 1 week and 2 weeks) after oral treatment of mice with lead nitrate when compared to controls. The same results were reported by Tewari et al., (2005), who observed a statistically significant increase in DNA damage in bone marrow cells from Swiss albino male mice exposed to leachates. Yuan and Tang (2001) studied the accumulation effect of lead acetate on DNA damage and the protection offered by selenium in mice blood cells for three generations. A significant induction of DNA damage was observed in both sexes of the second and third generations, suggesting that the accumulation effect of lead was very significant starting from the second generation. Valverde et al., (2001) explored the capacity of lead, cadmium or a mixture of both metals to interact with acellular DNA in cells from several organs of CD-1 mice by employing a variant of the comet assay. By means of this modified assay, that uses an enriched-lysis solution with proteinase-K and was described by Kasamatsu et al., (1996), DNA is no longer held under the regulation of any metabolic pathway or membrane barrier. They obtained a negative response in the induction of DNA damage in cells derived from the liver, kidney and lung. However, they observed the production of lipid peroxidation and an increase in free radical levels in the different organs after inhalation of lead acetate, suggesting the induction of genotoxicity and carcinogenicity by indirect interactions, such as oxidative stress.

Fish Studies

Despite no studies were reported employing SCE assay to evaluate genotoxic damage in fish exposed to lead, significant increases of cytogenetic alterations were found in lead-exposed fish by using CA test and MN assay. Ramsdorf et al., (2008) observed some little structural aberrations, such as gaps, in fish (*Hoplias malabaricus*) treated with different doses of lead nitrate by intraperitoneal injections, but the increase was not statistically significant. Also, Ferraro et al., (2004) found in the same fish treated orally with lead II a significant increase in the frequency of CA, but in this case the exposure time was higher than in Ramsdorf et al., (2008). Moreover, Taylor and Maher (2012) investigated the response of the fish *Anadara trapezia* to lead chloride spiked sediments. They observed that MN frequency significantly increased with exposure to increased lead concentrations. Also, Fatima et al., (2014) recently found increased levels of MN and DNA damage (evaluated by comet assay) in two fish species (*Channa striatus* and *Heteropneustes fossilis*) contaminated with different heavy metals including chromium, nickel and lead. In the same way, Harabay and Mosleh (2014), carried out a study to investigate the genotoxic and cytotoxic potentials of sublethal concentration (5mg/L) of combined metals (cadmium, copper, lead and zinc) on *Nile tilapia* erythrocytes after exposure for five and seven days. They found a significant increase in MN frequency after exposure to combined metals. However, similarly to Jacquet (1997) and Willems (1982) studies for mice and rabbits, respectively, Ramsdorf et al., (2008) and Monteiro et al., (2010) did not find any increase in the MN frequency when compared fish from a lead-exposed group with a control group. Ramsdorf et al., (2008) related their negative results to the low number of fish analyzed and to the fact that the piscine MN assay may lack sensitivity, since it does not detect the mitotic disjunctions if they do not provoke chromosomal loss in the anaphases neither chromosome aberrations caused by rearrangement, such as translocations or inversions if these do not originate acentric fragments (Metcalfe, 1989). Monteiro et al., (2010) attribute their negative results to the short time of exposure to lead, not enough to show MN.

The number of fish studies employing comet assay is considerably higher. Ramsdorf et al., (2008) evaluated the effects of inorganic lead in *H. malabaricus*. They found a significant difference between control and contaminated groups. Although differences among the applied doses were not observed, blood cells showed higher sensitivity than kidney cells, suggested to be caused by the acute contamination. There was one exception for kidney cells at the lowest dose, probably due to the short exposure time and also to the low quantity of lead, as the authors explained. These results are in agreement with Ferraro et al., (2004), who found a significant increase of tailed nucleoids in fish erythrocytes (*H. malabaricus*) treated with lead II, showing that extended exposures to lead contaminants are capable of originating damages in the genetic material of fish. Monteiro et al., (2010) also found that fish (*Prochilodus lineatus*) exposed to lead nitrate for 96 h showed a significant increase in the score of DNA damage in erythrocytes and liver cells when compared to respective controls, while gill cells showed a significant increase in DNA damage after 24 h and 96 h of exposure to lead. The authors attribute the increase of DNA damage only after 96 h of lead exposure in red blood cells and liver cells to the presence of metallothioneins (MT), cytosolic proteins of low molecular weight with the ability to bind to metal ions. MT synthesis may be determined by increased levels of metals in the body, preventing metal effects on DNA in shortest times of exposure. However, after 96 h of lead exposure, MT content returned to control levels, allowing lead to interact with intracellular compounds and cause DNA damage. Osman et al., (2008) used the alkaline comet assay for monitoring DNA strand breakage in sensitive early life stages of the African catfish *Clarias gariepinus* by exposure to lead nitrate at different concentrations and times of exposure. Strong correlations between increasing lead concentration, time of exposure and DNA strand breaks were observed.

Studies in Other Organisms

Several authors studied the effects of lead exposure on the genetic material of bean species (*Vicia faba*). Pourrut et al., (2011) and Shahid et al., (2011), for instance, studied the genotoxic effects of lead nitrate in *Vicia faba* roots, finding that MN frequencies were significantly higher in plants exposed to lead as compared to controls. Besides, they treated the plants with different concentrations of lead alone, and also with chelative agents (such as EDTA). When treated with both lead and EDTA, lead-induced MN frequency decreased significantly and in a dose dependent manner. Together with MN frequency, Pourrut et al., (2011) also studied the formation of DNA strand breaks caused by exposure of *Vicia faba* roots to lead nitrate. A significant increase in DNA fragmentation was found and the percentage of DNA in the comet tail correlated with lead concentration. Similarly, Lerda (1992) and later Kaur et al., (2014) found increases in genetic damage in *Allium cepa* exposed to lead by using CA test and comet assay, respectively.

Furthermore, significant increases of DNA damage with a direct dose-response pattern were observed after performing comet assay on larval hemocytes of *Drosophila melanogaster* treated with lead nitrate (Carmona et al., 2011).

2.3. Human Population Studies

Mutagenicity

Some epidemiological studies reported mutagenicity in subjects exposed to lead, both occupationally and environmentally. Van Larebeke et al., (2004) evaluated the differences in *hprt* mutant frequency in women residents in two Belgian industrial areas (Wilrijk and Hoboken) in association with blood lead levels. They observed a non-significant positive correlation in the *hprt* variant frequency in the total study population. Besides, their results showed that subjects with a blood lead concentration above the median tended to have higher *hprt* variant frequencies. These results agree with an indirect genotoxic effect of lead, as it was previously pointed.

Furthermore, there are a few studies which used the T-cell receptor (TCR) mutation assay to evaluate the potential genotoxic effects of human exposure to lead. T-cell receptor (TCR) is a heterodimer consisting of two peptide chains, α and β, which is expressed on the cell surface of the vast majority of peripheral T lymphocytes $CD4^+$ and $CD8^+$in association with CD3 molecule. The genes encoding for both chains are located on chromosomes 14 and 7, respectively, and they are phenotypically hemizygous. It is believed that only one of the TCR alleles is actively expressed as a result of an allelic exclusion mechanism similar to that observed in the immunoglobulin genes of B cells.

Therefore, it is expected that a single mutation in any of the TCR chains results in the absence of phenotypic expression of TCR on the cell surface (Kronenberg et al., 1986). Mutations in any of the TCR chain genes can be detected by means of flow cytometry using antibodies that recognize the CD3 molecule, because an incomplete TCR/CD3 complex cannot be transported to the cellular membrane. Some of the studies employing this technique for evaluation of genotoxic effects associated with lead exposure were carried out in our laboratory. We initially evaluated a population of 30 lead-exposed male workers (García-Lestón et al., 2008), in a second study 70 male workers were included (García-Lestón et al., 2011), and, in a third study a total of 148 male workers were analyzed (García-Lestón et al., 2012). Exposed individuals worked in two different factories engaged in the production of lead-acid batteries and glass chips, respectively. In all those studies, we found statistically significant differences between exposed and controls, showing the exposed groups higher TCR mutation frequencies than the control groups. Related to these results, Niu et al., (2015) observed significantly lower expression of TCR ζ-related factors, and *FcεRIγ* and *Elf-1* genes, which are involved in regulation of TCR expression, in 17 workers exposed to lead with regards to the control cases.

In contrast, Chen et al., (2006) did not observe significant differences between exposed and controls when they evaluated genotoxic effects of lead exposure in individuals from a workplace producing storage batteries. However, in this study the population size was smaller (25 exposed vs. 25 controls). Moreover, since the composition of both populations was statistically similar in terms of sex and tobacco smoking, the authors did not assess the impact of these factors on the results achieved, and they only focused on the evaluation of the differences between exposed and controls. Nevertheless, in the first studies the populations were different with regard to tobacco consumption, but not with regard to sex because all individuals were males, so the difference in the results could also be related to this fact.

Chromosome Alterations

In most studies assessing the genotoxic effects of lead in exposed people an increase in the frequency of SCE was observed (Bilban, 1998; Chen, 1992; Dönmez et al., 1998; Duydu et al., 2001; Duydu et al., 2005; Duydu and Süzen, 2003; Grandjean et al., 1983; Huang et al., 1988; Palus et al., 2003; Pinto et al., 2000; Rajah and Ahuja, 1995; Wiwanitkit et al., 2008; Wu et al., 2002; Wu et al., 2004). Moreover, in some of them a positive relationship between SCE frequency and blood lead levels (Bilban, 1998; Duydu et al.,

2001; Duydu and Süzen, 2003; Grandjean et al., 1983; Huang et al., 1988; Wiwanitkit et al., 2008; Wu et al., 2002) or between SCE rates and urinary lead concentrations (Chen, 1992) was found, whereas in other two works association with blood lead levels could not be observed (Dönmez et al., 1998; Pinto et al., 2000).

Nevertheless, some works reported no increase in the frequency of SCE in occupationally lead-exposed workers and in children environmentally exposed. Maki-Paakanen et al., (1981) analyzed SCE frequency in individuals exposed to lead in a smeltery and they did not find significant differences between the control group and the exposed group. However, they observed an increase in SCE rate in smoker exposed workers in comparison to smoker controls, similar than in Rajah and Ahuja (1995). This would indicate that tobacco smoke works as enhancer of the genotoxic effects of lead. Two other studies which assessed the effects of lead in children living in an extensively contaminated area (Dalpra et al., 1983; Myelzynska et al., 2006) did not show effect of the exposure on the frequency of SCE.

Given the results observed in epidemiological studies for CA test, there is considerable controversy regarding the ability of lead to cause chromosomal damage on exposed individuals. Several studies reported increases in the frequency of CA in human populations exposed to lead (Al-Hakkak et al., 1986; Bilban, 1998; Chen, 1992; Deknudt et al.,1973; Deknudt et al., 1977b; Deknudt and Leonard, 1975; Forni et al., 1976; Forni et al., 1980; Garza-Chapa et al., 1977; Grover et al., 2010; Hogstedt et al., 1979; Huang et al., 1988; Madhavi et al., 2008; Nordenson et al., 1978; Pinto et al., 2000; Piña-Calva et al., 1991; Sarto et al., 1978; Schwanitz et al., 1970; Schwanitz et al., 1975; Shaik and Jamil, 2009; Vaglenov et al., 1997). However, other works found no effects of lead exposure on CA frequencies (Bauchinger et al., 1972; Bauchinger et al., 1977; Bauchinger and Schmid, 1970; Bijlsma and de France, 1976; Horvat and Prpic-Majic, 1977; Maki-Paakkanen et al.,1981; Nordenson et al., 1982; O'Riordan and Evans, 1974; Pelclová et al.,1997; Schmid et al.,1972; Sperling et al., 1970). Moreover, Beckman et al., (1982) carried out a study in which CA frequencies in workers exposed to lead were evaluated at three different occasions (1976, 1978 and 1979). The results showed a significant increase of CA rates in lead-exposed workers in 1979, but not in 1976. But, after evaluating confounding factors, as smoking habits and simultaneous exposure to other toxic agents, the authors concluded that such variations in the frequency of CA could not be ascribed with certainty to changes in lead exposure.

Deknudt et al., (1977b) analyzed CA in cultured lymphocytes from two groups of lead-exposed people: workers from a smelting plant for storage batteries in Lyon (France) and workers from a factory of tin dishes in Nerem (Belgium). They found an increased number of severe aberrations (rings and dicentrics) in people from Lyon, whereas no such aberrations but an increased number of chromosome fragments were observed in those from Nerem. Furthermore, Huang et al., (1988) obtained mainly "light" CA (gaps, breaks, deletions and fragments) when the frequencies of CA in lead-exposed workers from a battery factory were analyzed, indicating minor lesions in the chromosomes.

Maki-Paakkanen et al., (1981) studied the frequency of CA in peripheral blood lymphocytes of workers exposed to lead in a smeltery. They found no significant differences in the CA rates between lead-exposed workers and unexposed controls. But, similar to Forni et al., (1980), they observed significantly higher rates of total aberrations in the 72 h culture regarding to the 50 h cultures. These results favor the previously proposed hypothesis (Forni and Secchi, 1973; Forni et al., 1976) that aberrations observed in lymphocyte cultures of lead-exposed subjects may be culture-born. This may be due to deficiency of repair functions in the presence of lead or some lead-induced metabolite which could accumulate with increasing culture time (Maki-Paakkanen et al., 1981).

Most epidemiological studies collected in the literature that use MN test to evaluate the potential genotoxic effects induced by exposure to lead are performed in individuals exposed in the workplace. In general, these studies could draw the conclusion that occupational exposure to lead causes genetic damage that, depending on the degree, could lead to cell unviability. To date, the vast majority of works showed an increase in the frequency of MN in individuals occupationally exposed to lead when compared with a control group. Minozzo et al., (2004) assessed the genetic damage in workers in the recycling of automotive batteries. They observed that both the concentrations of lead in blood and the frequency of MN in peripheral lymphocytes in the exposed group were significantly higher than in the control group. Moreover, the values of the nuclear division index (NDI) were significantly higher in the control group than in the exposed group, indicating a possible effect of lead on cell cycle. These results are consistent with other studies in individuals occupationally exposed to lead that showed an increase in the MN rate (Bilban, 1998; Chen et al., 2006; García-Lestón et al., 2012; Grover et al., 2010; Hamurcu et al., 2001; Kašuba et al., 2010; Kašubaet al., 2012; Martino-Roth et al., 2003; Minozzo et al., 2010; Palus et al., 2003; Pinto et al., 2000;

Shaik and Jamil, 2009; Vaglenov et al., 1998; Vaglenov et al., 2001; Wang et al., 2011).

Also, MN have been studied in exfoliated buccal epithelial cells. The buccal cell MN test is a minimally invasive method for studying DNA damage, chromosomal instability, cell death and the regenerative potential of human buccal mucosal tissue. For those reasons, the buccal MN test is increasingly used in molecular epidemiological studies in the last years. In their works, Grover et al., (2010), Khan et al., (2010) and Singh et al., (2013) observed an increase in the frequency of MN in individuals occupationally exposed to lead compared with a non-exposed control group.

The only epidemiological study that did not find positive effects of lead on the genetic material using the MN test was conducted by Hoffmann et al., (1984). They investigated the genotoxic effects in a group of car repair and radiator reconditioning workers, and they observed no significant differences between the exposed group and the control group. They had previously found a statistically significant correlation between "normal" blood lead values and CA in lymphocytes (Högstedt et al., 1979, 1981). But, according to the authors, the difference between these results could be explained either by the different cytogenetic methods employed or, more likely, by the fact that the earlier findings were due to a confounding exposure to other chemical substances with mutagenic potential.

Moreover, there is one study in the literature that was conducted in children environmentally exposed to complex mixtures including polycyclic aromatic hydrocarbons and lead (Mielzynska et al., 2006); in this work increases in the frequency of MN were obtained in the exposed children.

Primary DNA Damage

The comet assay has been used in many epidemiological studies as an important end-point to determine the possible induction of genotoxicity in individuals occupationally exposed to lead. Despite the controversy regarding the genotoxic properties of lead, most studies conducted to date in which DNA damage was assessed using the comet assay showed positive results.

Palus et al., (2003) assessed genotoxic damage in peripheral lymphocytes of workers from a Polish battery plant after high-level occupational exposure to lead and cadmium. The results of the comet assay showed a slightly but significantly increased rate in DNA migration compared to the control group. The same results were also reported in workers from battery plants by Fracasso et al., (2002), García-Lestón et al., (2012) and Restrepo et al., (2000), in secondary smelter lead workers (Steinmetz-Beck et al., 2005; Ye et al.,

1999;), in workers producing storage batteries and recycling of automotive batteries (Chen et al., 2006; Martino-Roth et al., 2003; Minozzo et al., 2010), in workers from a secondary lead recovery unit (Danadevi et al., 2003; Grover et al., 2010), in workers exposed to lead in ceramic industries (Kašuba et al., 2012), as well as in a study conducted in children environmentally exposed to lead (Méndez-Gómez et al., 2008).

The fact that most studies using the comet assay showed positive results, while other tests to assess genotoxic effects provided such different results, could be due to the different type of damage assessed, since the comet assay detects DNA damage that is quickly repaired and also the DNA repair processes that are taking place at the time of the experiment and are reflected as strand breaks in the assay.

However, García-Lestón et al., (2011) did not find significant differences between workers producing chemical substances and manufacturing lead-acid batteries and controls. These results may be related to the smaller sample size and to higher experimental variability in the other studies since, as the authors explained, they used a standardized comet assay in order to control for interassay variability.

DNA Repair

To the best of our knowledge, there is only one epidemiological study evaluating the effects of lead exposure on DNA repair systems. Al Bakheet et al., (2013) assessed the influence of long-term environmental human exposure to several heavy metals, including lead, on the expression of detoxifying, xenobiotic metabolizing, and DNA repair genes. They found that lead altered significantly the expression of several genes related to detoxification (*nqo1*, *ho-1*, *mt1*, *hsp70*) and xenobiotic metabolism (*cyp1a1*) processes, but not the mRNA expression of *ogg1* and *ape1*, genes, associated with DNA repair.

Conclusion

In this chapter, a number of toxicity studies, including *in vitro*, *in vivo* and epidemiological studies, evaluating the potential effects of lead on genetic material at different levels have been reviewed. Most of them reported that this heavy metal, in several different chemical forms, induce mutagenicity, chromosome alterations (especially SCE, CA and MN), DNA strand breaks and effects on DNA repair. However, some other studies showed different results. In the particular case of analysis of CA induction by lead chromate, several authors suggested that the increase found is mainly due to the toxic action of chromate and not to lead. In addition, several works did not report clear evidence on whether inorganic lead compounds exert clastogenic effects by themselves, or whether they enhance CA induced by compounds that occur simultaneously or arise during cell culturing (Beck and Obe, 1975; Deknudt and Leonard, 1975; Forni et al., 1980). Furthermore, some studies which did not find induction of SCE in workers occupationally exposed to lead showed increases in SCE rates in smoker exposed individuals, indicating that tobacco smoke works as enhancer of the genotoxic effects of lead (Maki-Paakanen, 1981; Rajah and Ahuja, 1995). This apparent inconsistency in the results may be due to the influence of some confounding factors including smoking habits, cell culturing time following the exposure, duration and route of lead exposure, and simultaneous exposure to other toxic agents that could influence the results.

Also, the type of cell evaluated in each work plays an important role in the interpretation of the data obtained, e.g., different types of cells could have different defense mechanisms against lead genotoxicity, as reported by Hwua and Yang (1998), suggesting that lead mutagenicity is positively correlated to the cellular oxidative stress. Furthermore, since most studies conducted in human populations employed blood cells and they remain in an arrested G0 phase (quiescent), any lesions induced in DNA may persist for some time (for instance, until cells are stimulated to divide in culture) (Winder and Bonin, 1993).

In addition to these possible reasons, the variability found in the studies evaluating lead genotoxicity may be also explained by the different action mechanisms showed by this metal. Indeed, it has been reported that effects of lead on genetic material could be due to indirect mechanisms (Garza et al., 2005; Hartwig et al., 1990; Hartwig, 1994; Kašubaet al., 2010; Landrigan et al., 2000; Silbergeld et al., 2003; Van Larebeke et al., 2004; Zhang et al., 2014). Lead can substitute calcium and/or zinc in processes and enzymes involved in DNA processing and repair, leading to inhibition of DNA repair and enhancement of genotoxicity when combined with other DNA damaging agents. Therefore, confounding factors as well as the indirect mechanisms of genotoxicity must be considered when assessing the genotoxic potential of lead compounds.

Acknowledgments

This work was funded by a grant from the Xunta de Galicia (GPC2013-058).

References

Aboul-Ela, E. I. (2002). The protective effect of calcium against genotoxicity of lead acetate administration on bone marrow and spermatocyte cells of mice in vivo. *Mutat. Res.516,* 1-9.

Aguilera, A. & Gómez-González, B. (2008). Genome instability: a mechanistic view of its causes and consequences. *Nat. Rev. Genet. 9*, 204-217.

Ahmad, A. & Shakoori, A. (2013). Cytotoxic and Genotoxic effects of Arsenic and Lead on Human Adipose Derived Mesenchymal Stem Cells (AMSCs). *J. Stem Cells Regen. Med. 9,* 29-36.

Al Bakheet, S. A., Attafi, I. M., Maayah, Z. H., Abd-Allah, A. R., Asiri, Y. A., Korashy, H. M. (2013). Effect of long-term human exposure to environmental heavy metals on the expression of detoxification and DNA repair genes. *Environ. Pollut. 181*, 226-232.

Albertini, R. J. & Hayes, R. B. (1997). Somatic cell mutations in cancer epidemiology. In: *Application of biomarkers in cancer epidemiology.* IARC Scientific Publications 142. Toniolo, P., Boffeta, P., Shuker, D. E. G, Rothman, N., Hulka, B. & Pearce, N. (Eds.). International Agency for Research on Cancer, Lyon. Pp. 159-184.

Albertini, R. J., Nicklas, J. A. & O'Neill, J. P. (1993). Somatic cell mutations in humans, biomarkers for genotoxicity. *Environ. Health Perspect.101* (Suppl. 3), 193-201.

Albertini, S. & Kirsch-Volders, M. (1997). Summary and conclusions on the MNT in vitro and application on testing strategies. *Mutat. Res.392,* 183-185.

Alghazal, M., Sutiakova, I., Kovalkovicova, N., Legath, J., Falis, M., Pistl, J., Sabo, R., Benova, K., Sabova, L. & Vaczi, P. (2008). Induction of micronuclei in rat bone marrow after chronic exposure to lead acetate trihydrate. *Toxicol Ind Health.24,* 587-593.

Al-Hakkak, Z. S., Hamamy, H. A., Murad, A. M. & Hussain, A. F. (1986). Chromosome aberrations in workers at a storage battery plant in Iraq. *Mutat Res.171,* 53-60.

Asakura, K., Satoh, H., Chiba, M., Okamoto, M., Serizawa, K., Nakano, M., Omae, K. (2009) Genotoxicity studies of heavy metals: lead, bismuth, indium, silver and antimony. *J. Occup. Health. 51*, 498-512.

Bauchinger, M., Dresp, J., Schmid, E., Englert, N. & Krause, C. (1977). Chromosome analyses of children after ecological lead exposure. *Mutat Res.56,* 75-80.

Bauchinger, M. & Schmid, E. (1970). Die cytogenetische wirkung von blei in menschlichen lymphozyten. *"Arbeitsgruppe Blei" der Kommission für Umveltgefahren des Bundesgesundheitsamtes, Berlin.*

Bauchinger, M. & Schmid, E. (1972). Chromosome analysis of cultures of Chinese hamster cells after treatment with lead acetate. *Mutat. Res.14,* 95-100.

Bauchinger, M., Schmid, E. & Schmid, D. (1972). Chromosomenanalyse bei Verkehrspolizisten mit erhöhter Bleilast. *Mutat. Res. 16,* 407-412.

Beckman, L., Nordenson, I. & Nordstrom, S. (1982). Occupational and environmental risks in and around a smelter in northern Sweden. VIII. Three-year follow-up of chromosomal aberrations in workers exposed to lead. *Hereditas.96,* 261-264.

Beek, B. & Obe, G. (1974). Effect of lead acetate on human leukocyte chromosomes in vitro. *Experientia.30,* 1006-1007.

Beek, B. & Obe, G. (1975). The human leukocyte test system. VI. The use of sister chromatid exchanges as possible indicators for mutagenic activities. *Humangenetik.29,* 127-134.

Bernstein, C. & Bernstein, H. (1991). *Aging, sex and DNA repair.* Academic Press USA, San Diego. Pp. 15-26.

Bihari, N., Batel, R. & Zahn, R. K. (1990). DNA damage determination by the alkaline elution technique in the haemolymph of mussel *Mytilus galloprovincialis* treated with benzo(a)pyrene and 4-nitroquinoline-N-oxide. *Aquat. Toxicol.18,* 13-22.

Bijlsma, J. B. & de France, H. F. (1976). Cytogenetic investigations in volunteers ingesting inorganic lead. *Int. Arch. Occup. Environ Health.38,* 145-148.

Bilban, M. (1998). Influence of the work environment in a Pb-Zn mine on the incidence of cytogenetic damage in miners. *Am. J. Ind. Med.34,* 455-463.

Bolognesi, C., Parrini, M., Roggieri, P., Ercolini, C. & Pellegrino, C. (1992). Carcinogenic and mutagenic pollutants: impact on marine organisms. In:

Proceedings of the FAO/UNEP/IOC workshop on the biological effects of pollutants onmarine organisms (Malta, September 10-14, 1991). MAP Technical Reports Series. *69,* 113-121.

Bolognesi, C., Rabboni, R. & Roggieri, P. (1996). Genotoxicity biomarkers in *Mytilus galloprovincialis*as indicators of marine pollutants. *Comp Biochem Physiol.113,* 319-323.

Bonacker, D., Stoiber, T., Bohm, K. J., Prots, I., Wang, M., Unger, E., Thier, R., Bolt, H. M. & Degen, G. H. (2005). Genotoxicity of inorganic lead salts and disturbance of microtubule function. *Environ. Mol. Mutagen. 45,* 346-353.

Bonassi, S., Znaor, A., Ceppi, M., Lando, C., Chang, W. P., Holland, N., Kirsch-Volders, M., Zeiger, E., Ban, S., Barale, R., Bigatti, M. P., Bolognesi, C., Cebulska-Wasilewska, A., Fabianova, E., Fucic, A., Hagmar, L., Joksic, G., Martelli, A., Migliore, L., Mirkova, E., Scarfi, M. R., Zijno, A., Norppa, H. & Fenech, M. (2007). An increased micronucleus frequency in peripheral blood lymphocytes predicts the risk of cancer in humans. *Carcinogenesis.28,* 625-631.

Cai, M. Y. & Arenaz, P. (1998). Antimutagenic effect of crown ethers on heavy metal-induced sister chromatid exchanges. *Mutagenesis.13,* 27-32.

Carmona, E. R., Creus, A., Marcos, R. (2011). Genotoxicity testing of two lead-compounds in somatic cells of Drosophila melanogaster. *Mutat. Res. 724,* 35-40.

Carrano, A. V. & Natarajan, A. T. (1988). Considerations for population monitoring using cytogenetic techniques. *Mutat. Res.204,* 379-406.

Cao, S., Duan, X., Zhao, X., Wang, B., Ma, J., Fanc, D., Sund, C., He, B., Wei, F., Jiang, G. (2015). Health risk assessment of various metal(loid)s via multiple exposure pathways on children living near a typical lead-acid battery plant, China. *Environ. Pollut. 200*, 16-23.

Celik, A., Ogenler, O. & Comelekoglu, U. (2005). The evaluation of micronucleus frequency by acridine orange fluorescent staining in peripheral blood of rats treated with lead acetate. *Mutagenesis.20,* 411-415.

Chen, Q. (1992). Lead concentrations in urine correlated with cytogenetic damage in workers exposed to lead. *Zhonghua Yu Fang Yi Xue Za Zhi. 26,* 334-335.

Chen, Z., Lou, J., Chen, S., Zheng, W., Wu, W., Jin, L., Deng, H. & He, J. (2006). Evaluating the genotoxic effects of workers exposed to lead using micronucleus assay, comet assay and TCR gene mutation test. *Toxicology.223,* 219-226.

Cole, J. & Skopek, T. R. (1994). ICPEMC Working Paper No. 3. Somatic mutant frequency, mutation rates and mutational spectra in the human population in vivo. *Mutat. Res.304,* 33-105.

Dalpra, L., Tibiletti, M. G., Nocera, G., Giulotto, P., Auriti, L., Carnelli, V. & Simoni, G. (1983). SCE analysis in children exposed to lead emission from a smelting plant. *Mutat. Res.120,* 249-256.

Danadevi, K., Rozati, R., Banu, B. S., Rao, P. H. & Grover, P. (2003). DNA damage in workers exposed to lead using comet assay. *Toxicology.187,* 183-193.

Deknudt, G., Colle, A. & Gerber, G. B. (1977a). Chromosomal abnormalities in lymphocytes from monkeys poisoned with lead. *Mutat. Res.45,* 77-83.

Deknudt, G. & Deminatti, M. (1978). Chromosome studies in human lymphocytes after in vitro exposure to metal salts. *Toxicology.10,* 67-75.

Deknudt, G. & Leonard, A. (1975). Cytogenetic investigations on leucocytes of workers from a cadmium plant. *Environ Physiol Biochem.5*, 319-327.

Deknudt, G., Manuel, Y. & Gerber, G. B. (1977b). Chromosomal aberrations in workers professionally exposed to lead. *J. Toxicol. Environ Health.3*, 885-891.

Deknudt, G. H., Leonard, A. & Ivanov, B. (1973). Chromosome aberrations observed in male workers occupationally exposed to lead. *Environ Physiol Biochem. 3*, 132-138.

Delile, H., Blichert-Toft, J., Goiran, J.P., Keay, S., Albarède, F. (2014). Lead in ancient Rome's city waters. *Proc. Natl. Acad. Sci. U S A. 111*, 6594-6599.

Devi, K. D., Banu, B. S., Grover, P. & Jamil, K. (2000). Genotoxic effect of lead nitrate on mice using SCGE (comet assay). *Toxicology.145,* 195-201.

Dhir, H., Roy, A. K. & Sharma, A. (1993). Relative efficiency of *Phyllanthus emblica* fruit extract and ascorbic acid in modifying lead and aluminium-induced sister-chromatid exchanges in mouse bone marrow. *Environ Mol. Mutagen.21,* 229-236.

Dönmez, H., Dursun, N., Ozkul, Y. & Demirtas, H. (1998). Increased sister chromatid exchanges in workers exposed to occupational lead and zinc. *Biol. Trace Elem. Res.61,* 105-109.

Douglas, G. R., Bell, R. D., Grant, C. E., Wytsma, J. M. & Bora, K. C. (1980). Effect of lead chromate on chromosome aberration, sister-chromatid exchange and DNA damage in mammalian cells in vitro. *Mutat. Res.77,* 157-163.

Duydu, Y., Dur, A., Süzen, H.S. (2005). Evaluation of increased proportion of cells with unusually high sister chromatid exchange counts as a cytogenetic biomarker for lead exposure. *Biol. Trace Elem. Res. 104*, 121-129.

Duydu, Y. & Süzen, H. S. (2003). Influence of delta-aminolevulinic acid dehydratase (ALAD) polymorphism on the frequency of sister chromatid exchange (SCE) and the number of high-frequency cells (HFCs) in lymphocytes from lead-exposed workers. *Mutat. Res. 540*, 79-88.

Duydu, Y., Süzen, H. S., Aydin, A., Cander, O., Uysal, H., Isimer, A. & Vural, N. (2001). Correlation between lead exposure indicators and sister chromatid exchange (SCE) frequencies in lymphocytes from inorganic lead exposed workers. *Arch. Environ. Contam. Toxicol.41,* 241-246.

Erickson, R.P. (2003). Somatic gene mutation and human disease other than cancer. *Mutat. Res. 543*, 125-136.

Fatima, M., Usmani, N., Mobarak Hossain. M., Siddiqui, M. F., Zafeer, M.F, Firdaus, F., Ahmad, S. (2014). Assessment of genotoxic induction and deterioration of fish quality in commercial species due to heavy-metal exposure in an urban reservoir. *Arch. Environ. Contam. Toxicol. 67*, 203-213. Ferraro, M. V., Fenocchio, A. S., Mantovani, M. S., Oliveira-Ribeiro, C. A. & Cestari, M. M. (2004). Mutagenic effects of lead (PbII) on the fish *H. malabaricus* as evaluated using the comet assay, piscine micronucleus and chromosome aberrations tests. *Genet. Mol. Biol. 27,* 103-107.

Forni, A., Cambiaghi, G. & Secchi, G. C. (1976). Initial occupational exposure to lead: Chromosome and biochemical findings. *Arch. Environ Health.31,* 73-78.

Forni, A., Sciame, A., Bertazzi, P. A. & Alessio, L. (1980). Chromosome and biochemical studies in women occupationally exposed to lead. *Arch Environ Health.35,* 139-146.

Forni, A. & Secchi, G. C. (1973). Chromosome changes in preclinical and clinical lead poisoning and correlation with biochemical findings. In: *International Symposium on Environmental Health Aspects of Lead* (Amsterdam). Barth, D., Berlin, A., Engel, R., Recht, P., Smeets, J. (Eds.). Commission of the European Communities, Luxembourg. Pp. 473-485.

Fracasso, M. E., Perbellini, L., Solda, S., Talamini, G. & Franceschetti, P. (2002). Lead induced DNA strand breaks in lymphocytes of exposed workers: role of reactive oxygen species and protein kinase C. *Mutat. Res.515,* 159-169.

Fu, H. & Boffetta, P. (1995). Cancer and occupational exposure to inorganic lead compounds: a meta-analysis of published data. *Occup. Environ Med. 52,* 73-81.

García-Lestón, J., Laffon, B., Roma-Torres, J., Teixeira, J. P., Monteiro, S., Pásaro, E., Prista, J., Mayan, O. & Méndez, J. (2008). Efectos genotóxicos e inmunotóxicos de la exposición laboral al plomo. *Arch. Prev. Riesgos. Labor.11,* 124-130.

García-Lestón, J., Roma-Torres, J., Vilares, M., Pinto, R., Cunha, L.M., Pristak, J., Teixeira, J.P., Mayan, O., Pásaro, E., Méndez, J., Laffon, B. (2011). Biomonitoring of a population of Portuguese workers exposed to lead. *Mutat. Res. 721*, 81-88.

García-Lestón, J., Roma-Torres, J., Vilares, M., Pinto, R., Prista, J., Teixeira, J.P., Mayan, O., Conde, J., Pingarilho, M., Gaspar, J.F., Pásaro, E., Méndez, J., Laffon, B. (2012). Genotoxic effects of occupational exposure to lead and influence of polymorphisms in genes involved in lead toxicokinetics and in DNA repair. *Environ. Int. 43*, 29-36.

Garza, A., Chávez, H., Vega, R. & Soto, E. (2005). Mecanismos celulares y moleculares de la neurotoxicidad por plomo. *Salud. Mental.28,* 48-58.

Garza-Chapa, R., Leal-Garza, C. H. & Molina-Ballesteros, G. (1977). Chromosome analysis in professional subjects exposed to lead contamination. *Arch. Invest. Med. (Mex).8*, 11-20.

Gasiorek, K. & Bauchinger, M. (1981). Chromosome changes in human lymphocytes after separate and combined treatment with divalent salts of lead, cadmium, and zinc. *Environ. Mutagen.3*, 513-518.

Gastaldo, J., Viau, M., Bencokova, Z., Joubert, A., Charvet, A. M., Balosso, J., Foray, N. (2007). Lead contamination results in late and slowly repairable DNA double-strand breaks and impacts upon the ATM-dependent signaling pathways. *Toxicol. Lett. 173*, 201–214.

Gerber, G. B., Léonard, A. & Jacquet, P. (1980). Toxicity, mutagenicity and teratogenicity of lead. *Mutat. Res.76,* 115-141.

Gadhia, S. R., Calabro, A. R., Barile, F. A. (2012). Trace metals alter DNA repair and histone modification pathways concurrently in mouse embryonic stem cells. *Toxicol. Lett. 212*, 169-179.

Goyer, R. A. & Rhyne, B. (1973). Pathological effects of lead. *Int. Rev. Exp. Pathol.12,* 1-77

Grandjean, P., Wulf, H. C. & Niebuhr, E. (1983). Sister chromatid exchange in response to variations in occupational lead exposure. *Environ Res. 32,* 199-204.

Grover, P., Rekhadevi, P.V., Danadevi, K., Vuyyuri, S.B., Mahboob, M., Rahman, M.F. (2010). Genotoxicity evaluation in workers occupationally exposed to lead. *Int. J. Hyg. Environ. Health. 213,* 99-106.

Gwini, S., MacFarlane, E., Del Monaco, A., McLean, D., Pisaniello, D., Benke, G. P., Sim, M. R. (2012). Cancer incidence, mortality, and blood lead levels among workers exposed to inorganic lead. *Ann. Epidemiol. 22*, 270-276.

Hamurcu, Z., Donmez, H., Saraymen, R. & Demirtas, H. (2001). Micronucleus frequencies in workers exposed to lead, zinc, and cadmium. *Biol Trace Elem Res.83,* 97-102.

Harabawy, A. S. & Mosleh, Y. Y. (2014). The role of vitamins A, C, E and selenium as antioxidants against genotoxicity and cytotoxicity of cadmium, copper, lead and zinc on erythrocytes of Nile tilapia, *Oreochromis niloticus*. *Ecotoxicol. Environ. Saf. 104*, 28-35.

Hartwig, A. (1994). Role of DNA repair inhibition in lead- and cadmium-induced genotoxicity: a review. *Environ. Health Perspect.102* (Suppl 3), 45-50.

Hartwig, A., Schlepegrell, R. & Beyersmann, D. (1990). Indirect mechanism of lead-induced genotoxicity in cultured mammalian cells. *Mutat. Res.241,* 75-82.

Hernberg, S. (2000). Lead poisoning in a historical perspective. *Am. J. Ind. Med.38,* 244-254.

Hoffmann, M., Hagberg, S., Karlsson, A., Nilsson, R., Ranstam, J. & Hogstedt, B. (1984). Inorganic lead exposure does not effect lymphocyte micronuclei in car radiator repair workers. *Hereditas.101,* 223-226.

Hogstedt, B., Kolnig, A. M., Mitelman, F. & Schutz, A. (1979). Correlation between blood-lead and chromosomal aberrations. *Lancet.2*, 262.

Horvat, D. J. & Prpic-Majic, D. (1977). Cytogenetic and biochemical study of lead exposed population. *Abstracts of the 2nd International Conference on Environmental Mutagen* (Edinburgh, England). P.174.

Huang, X. P., Feng, Z. Y., Zhai, W. L. & Xu, J. H. (1985). Chromosomal aberrations in the bone marrow cells of mice treated with lead acetic. *Occup. Health Chem. Ind. 2*, 7-9.

Huang, X. P., Feng, Z. Y., Zhai, W. L. & Xu, J. H. (1988). Chromosomal aberrations and sister chromatid exchanges in workers exposed to lead. *Biomed. Environ Sci.1*, 382-387.

Humphrey, R. M., Steward, D. L. & Sedita, B. A. (1968). DNA *Mutat. Res.6*, 459-465.

Hwua, Y. S. & Yang, J. L. (1998). Effect of 3-aminotriazole on anchorage independence and mutagenicity in cadmium- and lead-treated diploid human fibroblasts. *Carcinogenesis.19,* 881-888.

IARC (International Agency for Research on Cancer) (1987). IARC Monographs on the evaluation of carcinogenic risk to humans. Volumes 1 to 42. (Suppl. 7). *Overall evaluations of carcinogenicity: an updating of IARC monographs*. IARC, Lyon.

IARC (International Agency for Research on Cancer) (2006). IARC monographs on the evaluation of carcinogenic risks to humans. Volume 87. *Inorganic and organic lead compounds*.IARC, Lyon.

Jacquet, P., Leonard, A. & Gerber, G. B. (1977). Cytogenetic investigations on mice treated with lead. *J. Toxicol. Environ Health.2*, 619-624.

Jacquet, P. & Tachon, P. (1981). Effects of long-term lead exposure on monkey leukocyte chromosomes. *Toxicol. Lett.8*, 165-169.

Jagetia, G. C. & Aruna, R. (1998). Effect of various concentrations of lead nitrate on the induction of micronuclei in mouse bone marrow. *Mutat. Res.415,* 131-137.

Kasamatsu, T., Kohda, K. & Kawazoe, Y. (1996). Comparison of chemically induced DNA breakage in cellular and subcellular systems using the comet assay. *Mutat. Res.369,* 1-6.

Kašuba, V., Rozgaj, R., Milić, M., Zeljezić, D., Kopjar, N., Pizent, A., Kljaković-Gaspić, Z. (2010). Evaluation of lead exposure in battery-manufacturing workers with focus on different biomarkers. *J. Appl. Toxicol. 30,* 321-328.

Kašuba, V., Rozgaj, R., Milić, M., Zeljezić, D., Kopjar, N., Pizent, A., Kljaković-Gašpić, Z., Jazbec, A. (2012). Evaluation of genotoxic effects of lead in pottery-glaze workers using micronucleus assay, alkaline comet assay and DNA diffusion assay. *Int. Arch. Occup. Environ. Health. 85*, 807-818.

Kaur, G., Singh, H. P., Batish, D.R., Kohli, R. K. (2014) Pb-inhibited mitotic activity in onion roots involves DNA damage and disruption of oxidative metabolism. *Ecotoxicology. 23,* 1292-1304. Khan, M. I., Ahmad, I., Mahdi, A. A., Akhtar, M. J., Islam, N., Ashquin, M., Venkatesh, T. (2010). Elevated blood lead levels and cytogenetic markers in buccal epithelial cells of painters in India: genotoxicity in painters exposed to lead containing paints. Environ. *Sci. Pollut. Res. Int. 17*, 1347-1354.

Kohn, K. W., Erickson, L. C., Ewig, R. A. G. & Friedman, C. A. (1976). Fractionation of DNA from mammalian cells by alkaline elution. *Biochemistry. 15,* 4629-4637.

Kronenberg, M., Siu, G., Hood, L. E. & Shastri, N. (1986). The molecular genetics of the T-cell antigen receptor and T-cell antigen recognition. *Annu Rev Immunol.4*, 529-591.

Landrigan, P. J., Boffetta, P. & Apostoli, P. (2000). The reproductive toxicity and carcinogenicity of lead: A critical review. *Am. J. Ind. Med.38,* 231-243.

Lee, T. C. & Ho, I. C. (1995). Modulation of cellular antioxidant defense activities by sodium arsenite in human fibroblasts. *Arch. Toxicol.69,* 498-504.

Lerda, D. (1992). The effect of lead on *Allium cepa* L. *Mutat Res.281,* 89-92.

Li, R., Montpetit, A., Rousseau, M., Wu, S.Y., Greenwood, C.M., Spector, T.D., Pollak, M., Polychronakos, C., Richards, J.B. (2014). Somatic point mutations occurring early in development: a monozygotic twin study. *J. Med. Genet. 51*, 28-34.

Lin, C. J., Wu, K. H., Yew, F. H. & Lee, T. C. (1995). Differential cytotoxicity of cadmium to rat embryonic fibroblasts and human skin fibroblasts. *Toxicol. Appl. Pharmacol.133,* 20-26.

Lin, R. H., Lee, C. H., Chen, W. K. & Lin-Shiau, S. Y. (1994). Studies on cytotoxic and genotoxic effects of cadmium nitrate and lead nitrate in Chinese hamster ovary cells. *Environ. Mol. Mutagen.23,* 143-149.

Loi, S., Michiels, S., Lambrechts, D., Fumagalli, D., Claes, B., Kellokumpu-Lehtinen, P.L., Bono, P., Kataja, V., Piccart, M.J., Joensuu, H., Sotiriou C. (2013). Somatic mutation profiling and associations with prognosis and trastuzumab benefit in early breast cancer. *J. Natl. Cancer Inst. 105*, 960-967.

Lorencz, R., Nehéz, M. & Dési, I. (1996). Investigations on the mutagenic effects of cadmium and lead on the chromosomes of the bone marrow cells in subchronic experiments. In: *Abstracts of the XXVIIth Meeting of the Hungarian Society of Hygiene* (Blatonföldvár, Hungary, September 25-27).P. 116.

Madhavi, D., Devi, K. R. & Sowjanya, B. L. (2008). Increased frequency of chromosomal aberrations in industrial painters exposed to lead-based paints. *J Environ Pathol Toxicol Oncol.27,* 53-59.

Maki-Paakkanen, J., Sorsa, M. & Vainio, H. (1981). Chromosome aberrations and sister chromatid exchanges in lead-exposed workers. *Hereditas.94,* 269-275.

Martino-Roth, M. G., Viegas, J. & Roth, D. M. (2003). Occupational genotoxicity risk evaluation through the comet assay and the micronucleus test. *Genet. Mol. Res.2*, 410-417.

McBurney, M. W., Graham, F. L. & Whitmore, G. F. (1972). Sedimentation analysis of DNA from irradiated and unirradiated L-cells. *Biophys. J. 12,* 369-383.

McNeill, D.R., Wong, H.K., Narayana, A., Wilson, D.M. 3rd. (2007). Lead promotes abasic site accumulation and co-mutagenesis in mammalian cells by inhibiting the major abasic endonuclease Ape1. *Mol. Carcinog. 46*, 91-99.

Méndez-Gómez, J., Garcia-Vargas, G. G., Lopez-Carrillo, L., Calderon-Aranda, E. S., Gomez, A., Vera, E., Valverde, M., Cebrian, M. E. & Rojas, E. (2008). Genotoxic effects of environmental exposure to arsenic and lead on children in region Lagunera, Mexico. *Ann. N. Y. Acad. Sci. 1140,* 358-367.

Metcalfe, C. D. (1989). Testes for predicting carcinogenicity in fish. *CRC Cr Rev. Aquat. Sci. 1*, 111-129.

Mielzynska, D., Siwinska, E., Kapka, L., Szyfter, K., Knudsen, L. E. & Merlo, D. F. (2006). The influence of environmental exposure to complex mixtures including PAHs and lead on genotoxic effects in children living in Upper Silesia, Poland. *Mutagenesis.21,* 295-304.

Miller, B., Albertini, S., Locher, F., Thybaud, V. & Lorge, E. (1997). Comparative evaluation of the in vitro micronucleus test and the in vitro chromosome aberration test: industrial experience. *Mutat. Res.392,* 45-59.

Minozzo, R., Deimling, L. I., Gigante, L. P. & Santos-Mello, R. (2004). Micronuclei in peripheral blood lymphocytes of workers exposed to lead. *Mutat. Res.565,* 53-60.

Minozzo, R., Deimling, L. I., Santos-Mello, R. (2010). Cytokinesis-blocked micronucleus cytome and comet assays in peripheral blood lymphocytes of workers exposed to lead considering folate and vitamin B12 status. *Mutat. Res. 697*, 24-32.

Montaldi, A., Zentilin, L., Venier, P., Gola, I., Bianchi, V., Paglialunga, S. & Levis, A. G. (1985). Interaction of nitrilotriacetic acid with heavy metals in the induction of sister chromatid exchanges in cultured mammalian cells. *Environ. Mutagen.7*, 381-390.

Monteiro, V., Cavalcante, D.G., Viléla, M.B., Sofia, S.H, Martinez, C.B. (2010). In vivo and in vitro exposures for the evaluation of the genotoxic effects of lead on the Neotropical freshwater fish Prochilodus lineatus.*Aquat. Toxicol. 104*, 291-298.

Muro, L. A. & Goyer, R. A. (1969). Chromosome damage in experimental lead poisoning. *Arch Pathol.87,* 660-663.

Nayak, B. N., Ray, M., Persaud, T. V. & Nigli, M. (1989). Relationship of embryotoxicity to genotoxicity of lead nitrate in mice. *Exp. Pathol.36,* 65-73.

Needleman, H. (2004). Lead poisoning. *Annu. Rev. Med.* 55, 209–222

Niu, Y., Yu, W., Fang, S, Liu, S., Yang, Z., Liu, W., Chen, S., Yang, L., Li, B., Li, Y. (2015). Lead poisoning influences TCR-related gene expression patterns in peripheral blood T-lymphocytes of exposed workers. *J. Immunotoxicol. 12*, 92-97.

Nordenson, I., Beckman, G., Beckman, L. & Nordstrom, S. (1978). Occupational and environmental risks in and around a smelter in northern Sweden. IV. Chromosomal aberrations in workers exposed to lead. *Hereditas.88,* 263-267.

Nordenson, I., Nordstrom, S., Sweins, A. & Beckman, L. (1982). Chromosomal aberrations in lead-exposed workers. *Hereditas.96,* 265-268.

O'Riordan, M. L. & Evans, H. J. (1974). Absence of significant chromosome damage in males occupationally exposed to lead. *Nature. 247,* 50-53.

Olive, P. L. & Banath, J. P. (2006). The comet assay: a method to measure DNA damage in individual cells. *Nature Protocols.1*, 23-29.

Olive, P. L., Banath, J. P. & Durand, R. E. (1990). Heterogeneity in radiation-induced DNA damage and repair in tumour and normal cells measured using the "comet" assay. *Radiat Res.122,* 86-94.

Olive, P. L., Wledeck, D. & Banath, J. P. (1991). DNA double-strand breaks measured in individual cells subjected to gel electrophoresis. *Cancer Res.51,* 4671-4676.

Olsen, L. S., Nielsen, L. R., Nexo, B. A. & Wassermann, K. (1996). Somatic mutation detection in human biomonitoring. *Pharmacol. Toxicol.78,* 364-373.

Onalaja, A. O. & Claudio, L. (2000). Genetic susceptibility to lead poisoning. *Environ. Health Perspect.108* (Suppl 1), 23-28.

Osman, A. G., Mekkawy, I. A., Verreth, J., Wuertz, S., Kloas, W., Kirschbaum, F. (2008). Monitoring of DNA breakage in embryonic stages of the African catfish Clarias gariepinus (Burchell, 1822) after exposure to lead nitrate using alkaline comet assay.*Environ. Toxicol. 23*, 679-687.

Palus, J., Rydzynski, K., Dziubaltowska, E., Wyszynska, K., Natarajan, A. T. & Nilsson, R. (2003). Genotoxic effects of occupational exposure to lead and cadmium. *Mutat. Res.540,* 19-28.

Patierno, S. R., Banh, D. & Landolph, J. R. (1988). Transformation of C3H/10T1/2 mouse embryo cells to focus formation and anchorage independence by insoluble lead chromate but not soluble calcium chromate: relationship to mutagenesis and internalization of lead chromate particles. *Cancer Res.48,* 5280-5288.

Patierno, S. R. & Landolph, J. R. (1989). Soluble vs insoluble hexavalent chromate. Relationship of mutation to in vitro transformation and particle uptake. *Biol. Trace Elem. Res.21,* 469-474.

Patrick, L. (2006). Lead toxicity, a review of the literature. Part I: exposure, evaluation, and treatment. *Altern. Med. Rev.11,* 2-22.

Pelclová, D., Picková, J. & Patzelová, V. (1997). Chromosomal aberrations, hormone levels and oxidative phenotype (P450 2D6) in low occupational lead exposure. *Central Eur. J. Occup. Environ Med. 3*, 314-322.

Piao, F., Cheng, F., Chen, H., Li, G., Sun, X., Liu, S., Yamauchi, T. & Yokoyama, K. (2007). Effects of zinc coadministration on lead toxicities in rats. *Ind. Health.45,* 546-551.

Piña-Calva, A., Madrigal-Bujaidar, E., Fuentes, M. V., Neria, P., Perez-Lucio, C. & Velez-Zamora, N. M. (1991). Increased frequency of chromosomal aberrations in railroad car painters. *Arch. Environ Health.46,* 335-339.

Pinto, D., Ceballos, J. M., Garcia, G., Guzman, P., Del Razo, L. M., Vera, E., Gomez, H., Garcia, A. & Gonsebatt, M. E. (2000). Increased cytogenetic damage in outdoor painters. *Mutat. Res.467,* 105-111.

Poma, A., Pittaluga, E. & Tucci, A. (2003). Lead acetate genotoxicity on human melanoma cells in vitro. *Melanoma Res.13,* 563-566.

Pottier, G., Viau, M., Ricoul, M., Shim, G., Bellamy, M., Cuceu, C., Hempel, W. M., Sabatier, L. (2013). Lead exposure induces telomere instability in human cells. *PLoS One. 8*:e67501.

Pourrut, B., Jean, S., Silvestre, J., Pinelli, E. (2011). Lead-induced DNA damage in Vicia faba root cells: potential involvement of oxidative stress. *Mutat. Res. 726*, 123-128.

Rajah, T. & Ahuja, Y. R. (1995). In vivo genotoxic effects of smoking and occupational lead exposure in printing press workers. *Toxicol. Lett.76,* 71-75.

Rajaraman, P., Stewart, P.A., Samet, J.M., Schwartz, B.S., Linet, M.S., Zahm, S.H., Rothman, N., Yeager, M., Fine, H.A., Black, P.M., Loeffler, J., Shapiro, W.R., Selker, R.G., Inskip, P.D. (2006). Lead, genetic susceptibility, and risk of adult brain tumors. *Cancer Epidemiol. Biomarkers Prev. 15*, 2514-2520.

Ramsdorf, W. A., Ferraro, M. V., Oliveira-Ribeiro, C. A., Costa, J. R. & Cestari, M. M. (2008). Genotoxic evaluation of different doses of inorganic lead (PbII) in Hoplias malabaricus. *Environ Monit. Assess*. DOI 10.1007/s10661-008-0566-1.

Restrepo, H. G., Sicard, D. & Torres, M. M. (2000). DNA damage and repair in cells of lead exposed people. *Am. J. Ind. Med.38,* 330-334.

Robbiano, L., Carrozzino, R., Puglia, C. P., Corbu, C. & Brambilla, G. (1999). Correlation between induction of DNA fragmentation and micronuclei formation in kidney cells from rats and humans and tissue-specific carcinogenic activity. *Toxicol. Appl. Pharmacol. 161,* 153-159.

Robles-Osorio, M.L., & Sabath, E. (2014). Brief history of lead poisoning: from Egyptian civilization to the Renaissance. *Rev. Invest. Clin. 66*, 88-91.

Rojas, E., López, M. C. & Valverde, M. (1999). Single cell gel electrophoresis assay, methodology and applications. *J. Chromatogr. B.722,* 225-254.

Rydberg, B. (1975). The rate of strand separation in alkali of DNA of irradiated mammalian cells. *Radiat. Res. 61,* 274-287.

Sanders, T., Liu, Y. M., Tchounwou, P. B. (2014). Cytotoxic, genotoxic, and neurotoxic effects of Mg, Pb, and Fe on pheochromocytoma (PC-12) cells. *Environ. Toxicol.* doi: 10.1002/tox.22014.

Sandhu, S. S., Ma, T. H., Peng, Y. & Zhou, X. D. (1989). Clastogenicity evaluation of seven chemicals commonly found at hazardous industrial waste sites. *Mutat. Res.224,* 437-445.

Sarto, F., Stella, M. & Acqua, A. (1978). Cytogenetic study of a group of workers with increased lead absorption indices. *Med. Lav.69,* 172-180.

Schmid, E., Bauchinger, M., Pietruck, S. & Hall, G. (1972). Cytogenetic action of lead in human peripheral lymphocytes in vitro and in vivo. *Mutat. Res.16,* 401-406.

Schwanitz, G., Gebhart, E., Rott, H. D., Schaller, K. H., Essing, H. G., Lauer, O. & Prestele, H. (1975). Chromosome investigations in subjects with occupational lead exposure. *Dtsch Med. Wochenschr.100,* 1007-1011.

Schwanitz, G., Lehnert, G. & Gebhart, E. (1970). Chromosome damage after occupational exposure to lead. *Dtsch Med Wochenschr.95,* 1636-1641.

Shaik, A.P. & Jamil, K. (2009). Individual susceptibility and genotoxicity in workers exposed to hazardous materials like lead. *J. Hazard Mater. 168,* 918-924.

Shaik, A. P., Sankar, S., Reddy, S. C., Das, P. G. & Jamil, K. (2006). Lead-induced genotoxicity in lymphocytes from peripheral blood samples of humans: *in vitro* studies. *Drug Chem. Toxicol.1*, 111-124.

Sharma, R. K., Jacobson-Kram, D., Lemmon, M., Bakke, J., Galperin, I. & Blazak, W. F. (1985). Sister-chromatid exchange and cell replication kinetics in fetal and maternal cells after treatment with chemical teratogens. *Mutat. Res.158,* 217-231.

Silbergeld, E. K. (2003). Facilitative mechanisms of lead as a carcinogen. *Mutat. Res.533,* 121-133.

Silbergeld, E. K., Waalkes, M. & Rice, J. M. (2000). Lead as carcinogen: experimental evidence and mechanisms of action. *Am. J. Ind. Med.38,* 316-323.

Singh, N. P., McCoy, T., Tice, R. R. & Schneider, E. L. (1988). A simple technique for quantitation of low levels of DNA damage in individual cell. *Exp. Cell Res.175,* 184-192.

Singh, Z., Chadha, P., Sharma, S. (2013). Evaluation of oxidative stress and genotoxicity in battery manufacturing workers occupationally exposed to lead. *Toxicol. Int. 20*, 95-100.

Soltani, N., Keshavarzi, B., Moore, F., Tavakol, T., Lahijanzadeh, A.R., Jaafarzadeh, N., Kermani, M.. (2015). Ecological and human health hazards of heavy metals and polycyclic aromatic hydrocarbons (PAHs) in road dust of Isfahan metropolis, Iran. *Sci. Total Environ. 505*, 712-23.

Sperling, K., Weiss, G., Münzer, M. & Obe, G. (1970). Cromosomenuntersuchung an bleiexponierten Arbeitern. *"Arbeitsgruppe Blei" der Kommission für Umveltgefahren des Bundesgesundheitsamtes, Berlin.*

Steinert, S. A., Streib-Moutee, R., Leather, J. M. & Chadwick, D. B. (1998). DNA damage in mussels at sites in San Diego Bay.*Mutat Res.399,* 65-85.

Steinmetz-Beck, A., Szahidewicz-Krupska, E., Beck, B., Poreba, R. & Andrzejak, R. (2005). Genotoxicity effect of chronic lead exposure assessed using the comet assay. *Med. Pr.56,* 295-302.

Tachi, K., Nishimae, S. & Saito, K. (1985). Cytogenetic effects of lead acetate on rat bone marrow cells. *Arch. Environ Health.40,* 144-147.

Taningher, M., Bordone, R., Russo, P., Santi, L. & Carlone, S. (1987). Major discrepancies between results obtained with two different methods for evaluating DNA damage: Alkaline elution and alkaline unwinding. Posible explanations. *Anticancer. Res.7*, 669-680.

Taylor, A.M. & Maher, W.A. (2012). Exposure-dose-response of Anadara trapezia to metal contaminated estuarine sediments. 2. Lead spiked sediments. *Aquat. Toxicol. 116-117*, 79-89.

Tewari, A., Chauhan, L. K., Kumar, D. & Gupta, S. K. (2005). Municipal sludge leachate-induced genotoxicity in mice – a subacute study. *Mutat Res.587,* 9-15.

Thier, R., Bonacker, D., Stoiber, T., Bohm, K. J., Wang, M., Unger, E., Bolt, H. M. & Degen, G. (2003). Interaction of metal salts with cytoskeletal motor protein systems. *Toxicol Lett.140-141,* 75-81.

Thornton, I., Rautiu, R., Bush, S.M. (2001) Lead the facts. IC Consultants Ltd. London, UK

Tice, R. R. (1995). The single cell gel/comet assay: a microgel electrophoretic technique for the detection of DNA damage and repair in individual cells. In, *Environmental Mutagenesis*. Bios Scientific Publishers, Oxford. Pp. 315-339.

Tice, R. R., Agurell, E., Anderson, D., Burlinson, B., Hartmann, A., Kobayashi, H., Miyamae, Y., Rojas, E., Ryu, J. C. & Sasaki, Y. F. (2000). Single cell gel/comet assay: guidelines for in vitro and in vivo genetic toxicology testing. *Environ. Mol. Mutagen.35,* 206-221.

Todd, A. C., Wtmur, J. G., Moline, J. M., Godbold, J. H., Levin S. H. & Landrigan, P. J. (1996). Unraveling the chronic toxicity of lead: An essential priority for environmental health. *Environ Health Perspect. 104,* 141-146.

Tapisso, J., Marques, C.C., Mathias, M.da L., Ramalhinho, M.da G. (2009). Induction of micronuclei and sister chromatid exchange in bone-marrow cells and abnormalities in sperm of Algerian mice (Mus spretus) exposed to cadmium, lead and zinc. *Mutat. Res. 678,* 59-64.

Vaglenov, A., Carbonell, E. & Marcos, R. (1998). Biomonitoring of workers exposed to lead. Genotoxic effects, its modulation by polyvitamin treatment and evaluation of the induced radioresistance. *Mutat. Res.418,* 79-92.

Vaglenov, A., Creus, A., Laltchev, S., Petkova, V., Pavlova, S. & Marcos, R. (2001). Occupational exposure to lead and induction of genetic damage. *Environ Health Perspect.109,* 295-298.

Vaglenov, A. K., Laltchev, S. G., Nosko, M. S. & Pavlova, S. P. (1997). Cytogenetic monitoring of workers exposed to lead. *Cent. Eur. J. Occup. Environ Med. 3,* 298-308.

Valverde, M., Fortoul, T. I., Diaz-Barriga, F., Mejia, J. & del Castillo, E. R. (2002). Genotoxicity induced in CD-1 mice by inhaled lead: differential organ response. *Mutagenesis.17,* 55-61.

Valverde, M., Trejo, C. & Rojas, E. (2001). Is the capacity of lead acetate and cadmium chloride to induce genotoxic damage due to direct DNA-metal interaction? *Mutagenesis.16,* 265-270.

Van Larebeke, N., Koppen, G., Nelen, V., Schoeters, G., Van Loon, H., Albering, H., Riga, L., Vlietinck, R., Kleinjans, J. (2004). Differences in HPRT mutant frequency among middle-aged Flemish women in association with area of residence and blood lead levels. *Biomarkers. 9,* 71-84.

Veatch, W. &Okada, S. (1969). Radiation-induced breaks of DNA in cultured mammalian cells. *Biophys J. 9*, 330-346.

Vukmirovic, M., Bihari, N., Zahn, R. K., Müller, W. E. G. & Batel, R. (1994). DNA damage in marine mussel *Mytilusgalloprovincialis* as a biomarker of environmental contamination. *Mar. Ecol. Prog Ser. 109,* 165-171.

Wang, Q., He, . AM., Gao, B., Chen, L., Yu, Q. Z., Guo, H., Shi, B. J., Jiang, P., Zhang, Z. Y, Li, P. L., Sheng, Y. G., Fu, M. J., Wu, C. T., Chen, M. X., Yuan, J. (2011). Increased levels of lead in the blood and frequencies of lymphocytic micronucleated binucleated cells among workers from an electronic-waste recycling site. *J. Environ. Sci. Health A. Tox. Hazard Subst. Environ. Eng. 46,* 669-676.

Wedeen, R.P. (2011). Lead poisoning: the evolving definition. *Int. J. Occup. Environ. Med. 2*, 1-3.

Wilhelm, M., Heinzow, B., Angerer, J., Schulz, C. (2010). Reassessment of critical lead effects by the German Human Biomonitoring Commission results in suspension of the human biomonitoring values (HBM I and HBM II) for lead in blood of children and adults. *Int. J. Hyg. Environ. Health. 213*, 265-269.

Willems, M. I., de Schepper, G. G., Wibowo, A. A., Immel, H. R., Dietrich, A. J. & Zielhuis, R. L. (1982). Absence of an effect of lead acetate on sperm morphology, sister chromatid exchanges or on micronuclei formation in rabbits. *Arch. Toxicol.50,* 149-157.

Wilson, J. T., Pascoe, P. L., Parry, J. M. & Dixon, D. R., (1998). Evaluation of the comet assay as a method for the detection of DNA damage in the cells of a marine invertebrate *Mytilusedulis* L. (Mollusca: Pelecypoda). *Mutat. Res.399,* 87-95.

Winder, C. & Bonin, T. (1993). The genotoxicity of lead. *Mutat. Res.285,* 117-124.

Wise, J. P., Leonard, J. C. & Patierno, S. R. (1992). Clastogenicity of lead chromate particles in hamster and human cells. *Mutat Res.278,* 69-79.

Wise, J. P., Sr., Stearns, D. M., Wetterhahn, K. E. & Patierno, S. R. (1994). Cell-enhanced dissolution of carcinogenic lead chromate particles: the role of individual dissolution products in clastogenesis. *Carcinogenesis.15,* 2249-2254.

Wise, S. S., Schuler, J. H., Holmes, A. L., Katsifis, S. P., Ketterer, M. E., Hartsock, W. J., Zheng, T. & Wise, J. P., Sr. (2004). Comparison of two particulate hexavalent chromium compounds, Barium chromate is more genotoxic than lead chromate in human lung cells. *Environ Mol. Mutagen.44,* 156-162.

Wise, S. S., Schuler, J. H., Katsifis, S. P. & Wise, J. P., Sr. (2003). Barium chromate is cytotoxic and genotoxic to human lung cells. *Environ Mol. Mutagen.42,* 274-278.

Wiwanitkit, V., Suwansaksri, J. & Soogarun, S. (2008). White blood cell sister chromatid exchange among a sample of Thai subjects exposed to lead: Lead-induced genotoxicity. *Toxicol. Environ. Chem. 90,* 765-768.

Wozniak, K. & Blasiak, J. (2003). In vitro genotoxicity of lead acetate, induction of single and double DNA strand breaks and DNA-protein cross-links. *Mutat. Res.535,* 127-139.

Wu, F. Y., Chang, P. W., Wu, C. C. & Kuo, H. W. (2002). Correlations of blood lead with DNA-protein cross-links and sister chromatid exchanges in lead workers. *Cancer Epidemiol. Biomarkers Prev.11,* 287-290.

Wu, F. Y., Chang, P. W., Wu, C. C., Lai, J.S., Kuo, H. W. (2004). Lack of association of delta-aminolevulinic acid dehydratase genotype with cytogenetic damage in lead workers. *Int. Arch. Occup. Environ. Health. 77*, 395-400.

Wulf, H. C. (1980). Sister chromatid exchanges in human lymphocytes exposed to nickel and lead. *Dan. Med. Bull. 27,* 40-42.

Xie, H., Wise, S. S., Holmes, A. L., Xu, B., Wakeman, T. P., Pelsue, S. C., Singh, N. P. & Wise, J. P., Sr. (2005). Carcinogenic lead chromate induces DNA double-strand breaks in human lung cells. *Mutat. Res.586,* 160-172.

Xu, J., Wise, J. P., Patierno, S. R. (1992). DNA damage induced by carcinogenic lead chromate particles in cultured mammalian cells. *Mutat. Res.280,* 129-136.

Yang, J. L., Yeh, S. C. & Chang, C. Y. (1996). Lead acetate mutagenicity and mutational spectrum in the hypoxanthine guanine phosphoribosyltransferase gene of Chinese hamster ovary K1 cells. *Mol Carcinog.17,* 181-191.

Ye, X. B., Fu, H., Zhu, J. L., Ni, W. M., Lu, Y. W., Kuang, X. Y., Yang, S. L. & Shu, B. X. (1999). A study on oxidative stress in lead-exposed workers. *J. Toxicol. Environ. Health A.57,* 161-172.

Yuan, X. & Tang, C. (2001). The accumulation effect of lead on DNA damage in mice blood cells of three generations and the protection of selenium. *J. Environ. Sci. Health A Tox. Hazard Subst. Environ. Eng.36,* 501-508.

Zhang, H., Wei, K., Zhang, M., Liu, R., Chen, Y. (2014). Assessing the mechanism of DNA damage induced by lead through direct and indirect interactions. *J. Photochem. Photobiol. B. 136*, 46-53.

Zelikoff, J. T. & Li, J. H., Hartwig, A., Wang, X. W., Costa, M., Rossman, T. G. (1988). Genetic toxicology of lead compounds. *Carcinogenesis.9*, 1727-1732.

In: Lead Exposure and Poisoning
Editor: Leonard Horton
ISBN: 978-1-63482-699-0

Chapter II

Health Risk Assessment of Environmental Lead Exposures Through Scrapped Car Paint Dusts from Fairly Used Car Painting Workshops in Nigeria

John Kanayochukwu Nduka[1*], Johnpaul Onyenezi Amuka[1] and John Friday Sale[2]

[1] Environmental Chemistry and Toxicology Research Unit, Pure and Industrial Chemistry Department, Nnamdi Azikiwe University. Awka. Anambra State. Nigeria

[2] Department of Chemistry, Kogi State University, Kogi State. Nigeria

Abstract

Background: High volume of automobiles imported into Nigeria are fairly used. Due to the resultant effect of the high rate of road accidents and ambient air temperature which cause expansion and contraction on these vehicles, they undergo wear and tear as could be seen by the caking

* johnnduka2000@yahoo.co.uk, +234- 7039541583

and flaking of the paint coatings. The vehicles are then taken to the car painting workshops for reworking (scrapping and repainting).

Method: About fifty-six (56) scrapped paint dusts from 56 vehicles were collected from eight (8) different car paint workshops in south eastern Nigerian. They were homogenized, mixed and divided into fine particles that can pass through 0.5mm sieve and digested by standard method. The filtrates were assayed with atomic absorption spectrophotometry (AAS 200A).

Results: Show that the lead (Pb) concentration were in the range of (1.42 ± 0.01 - 4.16 ± 0.01mg/kg) for workshop 1, (0.49 ± 0.01-3.50 ± 0.01mg/kg) for workshop2, (2.45 ± 0.01-4.36 ± 0.04mg/kg) for workshop 3, (2.94 ± 0.02-4.17 ± 0.00mg/kg) for workshop 4, etc; Dose exposure and risk assessment through inhalation and dermal contact were below USA EPA threshold limit.

Conclusion: Reworking (scrapping and repainting) of fairly used vehicles imported into Nigeria may contribute to environmental lead burden with its associated public health risks.

Keywords: health risk assessment, lead exposure, automobile paint dust, fairly used and worn out vehicles, environmental pollution

Introduction

Galena (PbS) is the major ore containing lead. Main producers are Russia (17%), Australia (14%), USA (10%), Canada (9%), Peru, Mexico and China (6%) each. Total world production of lead from PbS stood at 3.1 million tonnes in 1992. More than 55% of lead produced in 1985 was utilized in making lead/acid car battery. Lead and lead compounds were also used as additives in petrol, paints, lead pipes and solder, and also in rust proofing metals and corrugated steel (Lee, 1996).

In recent years, the use of lead in these products has declined markedly because of its toxicity. The implication of this is that lead as a metal, associated with human activities for decades, has been a common industrial metal wide spread in air, water, dust, soil, and food.

Projenitors of civilization have included lead in the manufacture of home utensils, jugs, trays and decorative articles. A compilation has been made of 120 occupations e.g. auto-mechanic, painting, printing, welding etc. that involves exposure to lead (Wallace and Cooper, 1986). A consequence of this is that lead is widely distributed in the environment today. It has been established that all humans have lead in their bodies, primarily as a result of exposure to man-made sources (ATSDR, 1992). This is possible because consumable products are laden with chemical elements, this is of interest because they are either essential or toxic in nature (Onianwa et al., 1999), non-consumable goods also contain approximately high amount of chemical element. Lead is present in food and drinking water and high especially if the water is soft, acidic and is distributed in lead pipelines, meaning that the primary route of exposure to lead is through drinking water from lead-based plumbing materials (US EPA, 1989). Other economic or occupational activities that may lead to lead exposure in adults include industrial activities like mining, smelting, refining and manufacturing processes and earth works such as road construction. In children, lead poisoning may result from ingestion of lead in flaking lead paints in old houses (Nduka et al., 2008), in lead containing objects and in contaminated food (Bruening et al., 1999), as well as in commonly administered pediatric syrups (Orisakwe and Nduka, 2009). Dairy products which are important components of children's diet (Fakayode and Olu-Owolabi, 2003), canned and non-canned beverages (Maduabuchi et al., 2006), as well as herbal preparations (Obi et al., 2006), are also exposure pathways of lead poisoning. The environmental routes of lead (Pb) exposure in Nigeria are as varied as its toxicity to humans. Most studies in Nigeria have tended to portray automobile emissions as the only major source of lead exposure (Kakulu, 2003, Nduka and Orisakwe, 2010). This notion was due to the fact that before now, organic lead compounds (tetraethyl lead and tetramethyl lead) were extensively used as additives in gasoline but at present unleaded gasoline used in most countries of the world and Africa including Nigeria has contributed substantially to global lead pollution (Nriagu, 1978, 1979, 1989; Anon, 1996). Despite global effort on reduction or outright non inclusion of lead in gasoline, that with an average lead content of 0.66g/L remains in use in Nigeria as at 2003 (Fakayode and Olu-Owolabi, 2003b).

Studies has also shown that fairly used electronics such as computers and its accessories, TV sets, fax machines, cell phones, telephones, photocopy machines and printers, dryers, wireless devices, video cameras, chips, motherboards, cathode ray tubes and peripheral items, kitchen equipments, electronic toys, washing machines, refrigerators etc. are veritable sources of lead exposure in Nigeria and indeed Africa. Because of the fact that large volumes of these materials imported into the country are irreparable junk which the country lacks the technology to safely dispose, more than 75% of them wind up in landfills and informal dumps that dot the Nigerian landscape where they decompose and release toxic metals such as lead into the environment (Schmidt, 2006; Orisakwe and Frazzoli, 2010; Frazzoli et al., 2010). The irony is that most modern cars/vehicles are fitted with some of these electronic devices. Even some mechanical components of vehicles/cars are made of metals and metalloids that contain arsenic, cadmium, chromium, copper, lead and mercury and organic chemicals such as brominated flame retardants (BFRs). Since the automobile industry/trade like electronics is another sector that is associated with high volume of importation into Nigeria from Europe, America and some Asian tigers, there are concerns that toxic chemicals will leach from electronic and mechanical devices when disposed (White et al., 2003). It has been adduced that Nigerians patronize fairly used (second hand) vehicles with very short life span because of poverty. High percentage of these vehicles and their parts are worn-out, rickety and no longer road worthy and with an alarming rate of vehicular road accident in Nigeria coupled with deplorable road conditions, and high ambient air temperature that cause expansion and contraction, the net effect is that the vehicles are taken to the workshops where they are re-worked (paints are scrapped and repainted).

Based on the above impressions, this work is simply to show that scrapping and repainting of rickety old vehicles add to environmental lead burden in Nigeria as we are not aware of any work disposed on that. We are not aware of any manuscript on metal exposure through automobile paint dust in Nigeria, hence this works, which is simply to show that scrapping and repainting of rickety old vehicles add to environmental lead burden in Nigeria.

Materials and Methods

We used drive-by exercise to identify panel beating/automobile paint workshops with beehive of activities, where a total of eight (8) in numbers were identified. Through friendly discussion and explanation, we were allowed to collect scrapped paint dust with white cardboard sheets from a number of available vehicles as at the time of the visits. The paint matrixes were stored in black polythene bags before digestion and analysis. They were ground, mixed and divided into fine particles that could pass through a 0.5mm sieve. Digestion was done by placing 2g of paint dust in a conical flask, adding 15ml of concentrated nitric acid and perchloric acid at a ratio 1:1 and heating in a fume cupboard at a temperature of 105°C until the volume went down to less than 1ML, it was allowed to cool, 10ML of de-ionized water were added then stirred and filtered and made up in standard volumetric flask. Lead metal was assayed with atomic absorption spectrophotometry (AAS 200A) with a detection limit for Pb set at 0.001mg/L, with blank values reading as 0.00mg/L in de-ionized water with electrical conductivity value of lower than 5μs/cm. Samples were analysed in triplicates and results shown in Table 1 reported in SD and Mean ± SEM.

Exposure and Risk Assessment Method

The model employed in this study is that developed by the US Environmental Protection Agency (US Environmental Protection Agency, 1996) and the Dutch National Institute of Public Health and Environmental Protection (Van den Berg, 1995). A worker at an automobile workshop (engaged in scrapping old and worn out car paints and repainting or any other ancillary or support work) may be exposed to lead poisoning through inhalation or dermal contact. If children are involved or proper hygiene is not observed by the workers exposure through ingestion may be possible, but we are restricting our study to adults. Exposure is expressed in terms of a daily dose and is calculated separately for each vehicle for a given exposure pathway. The doses contacted through dermal contact (dose absorbed through the skin) and inhalations of the scrapped paint dust were calculated using the equations (1&2) below (adapted from US Environmental Protection Agency, 1996).

$$D_{inh}\,(mgkg^{-1}day^{-1}) = C\,(mgkg^{-1}) \times \frac{InhR \times EF \times ED}{PEF \times BW \times AT} \longrightarrow \quad (1)$$

Dose absorbed through dermal contact with scrapped paint dust particles,

$$D_{dermal}\,(mgkg^{-1}day^{-1}) = C\,(mgkg^{-1}) \times \frac{SA \times SL \times ABS \times EF \times ED \times 10^{-6}}{BW \times AT} \longrightarrow \quad (2)$$

Where C is the concentration of lead (Pb) in scrapped paint dust matrix (exposure point concentration) at the workshop (shown in Table 1), InhR is the inhalation rate. In this study, we are adopting Inh R = $7.6m^3day^{-1}$ (Van den Berg, 1995). EF the exposure frequency, in this study, EF = 180day yr^{-1} (workshop specific). ED the exposure duration, in this study, ED = 6yrs (workshop specific). SA the exposed skin area, in this study, SA = $2800cm^2$

(US Environmental Protection Agency, 2001). SL is the skin adherence factor, in this study, SL = $0.2 mgcm^{-2}day^{-1}$ (US Environmental Protection Agency, 2001). ABS the dermal absorption factor (unit less), in this study, ABS = 0.001 (US Department of Energy, 2004). PEF the particle emission factor, in this study, PEF = $1.36 \times 10^9 m^3 kg^{-1}$ (US Environmental Protection Agency, 2001). BW the average body weight, in this study, BW = 15kg (US Environmental Protection Agency, 1989) and AT the average time for lead (a non carcinogen), AT (days) = ED x 365. Results of lead exposure through inhalation and dermal contact calculated using equation 1 and 2 were presented in Table 2.

The non-carcinogenic risk from lead metals can be expressed as the hazard quotient.

$$HQ = (CDI(E))/RFD \longrightarrow \quad (3)$$

'CDI (E)' is the chronic daily intake (exposure) and 'RFD' is the chronic reference dose of the lead ($mg\ kg^{-1}d^{-1}$) (Liu et al., 2013). The results are shown in Table 3.

$$\text{Chronic hazard index} = \sum_{k=1}^{n} CDI(E)\kappa/RFD \longrightarrow$$

where the chronic hazard index (HI) is the sum of more than one hazard quotient for multiple substances or multiple exposure pathways. In this study, exposure is through different vehicles in different workshops and two exposure pathways (inhalation and dermal contact). The results is shown in Table 4 (Liu et al., 2013)

Results

Table 1 shows the lead concentration in paint dust matrix from each of the seven (7) vehicles in all the eight (8) workshop of study (workshop eight has six vehicles). The results ranged from 2.12 ± 0.03 – 4.04 ± 0.09 (workshop 1), 3.08 ± 0.01 – 5.55 ± 0.03 (workshop 2), 2.45 ± 0.01 – 3.17 ± 0.00 (workshop 3), 2.45 ± 0.01 – 4.36 ± 0.04 (workshop 4) … 2.30 ± 0.08 – 3.17 ± 0.00 (workshop 8). All the scrapped paint dust matrix from each of the vehicles in all the workshops were in the concentration that can contribute to environmental lead burden and constitute health risk to humans.

Table 1. Shows the concentration of lead in scrapped car paint dust of different vehicles at different workshops

S/N	Workshop	Data	Vehicle 1	Vehicle 2	Vehicle 3	Vehicle 4	Vehicle 5	Vehicle 6	Vehicle 7
	1	SD Mean ± SEM	0.24 3.33 ± 0.14	0.02 4.04 ± 0.09	0.04 3.75 ± 0.02	0.02 3.88 ± 0.01	0.06 2.12 ± 0.03	0.01 2.17 ± 0.01	0.04 2.43 ± 0.02
	2	SD Mean ± SEM	0.01 4.62 ± 0.10	0.03 3.08 ± 0.01	0.04 3.44 ± 0.02	0.02 3.38 ± 0.01	0.01 4.01 ± 0.01	0.06 5.55 ± 0.03	0.04 5.41 ± 0.02
	3	SD Mean ± SEM	0.03 2.48 ± 0.02	0.03 2.81 ± 0.02	0.09 2.63 ± 0.05	0.02 2.45 ± 0.01	0.11 2.52 ± 0.64	0.01 3.17 ± 0.00	0.01 2.93 ± 0.00
	4	SD Mean ± SEM	0.06 4.36 ± 0.04	0.05 3.99 ± 0.03	0.01 4.17 ± 0.00	0.02 3.41 ± 0.01	0.03 2.94 ± 0.02	0.01 3.17 ± 0.01	0.02 3.50 ± 0.01
	5	SD Mean ± SEM	0.02 3.09 ± 0.01	0.01 2.16 ± 0.01	0.01 1.17 ± 0.01	0.01 0.93 ± 0.01	0.02 0.49 ± 0.01	0.04 2.12 ± 0.02	0.02 3.50 ± 0.01
	6	SD Mean ± SEM	0.02 2.45 ± 0.01	0.01 2.03 ± 0.01	0.01 3.17 ± 0.01	0.02 6.30 ± 0.01	0.01 4.15 ± 0.01	0.01 2.98 ± 0.01	0.01 3.11 ± 0.00
	7	SD Mean ± SEM	0.02 4.16 ± 0.01	0.01 4.16 ± 0.01	0.03 2.40 ± 0.02	0.01 1.42 ± 0.01	0.02 2.05 ± 0.01	0.01 2.02 ± 0.01	0.02 3.76 ± 0.01
	8	SD Mean ± SEM	0.02 2.92 ± 0.01	0.01 2.72 ± 0.01	0.01 3.17 ± 0.00	0.01 2.93 ± 0.00	0.02 3.11 ± 0.00	0.14 2.30 ± 0.08	—

(n = 3).

Table 2. Shows lead dose contacted through inhalation and dermal contact with scrapped car paint dust

S/N	Workshop	Vehicle 1	Vehicle 2	Vehicle 3	Vehicle 4	Vehicle 5	Vehicle 6	Vehicle 7
	1	5.244E-11 (5.255E-9)	6.362E-11 (6.376E-9)	5.905E-11 (5.918E-9)	5.323E-11 (5.918E-9)	3.339E-11 (3.346E-9)	3.417E-11 (3.424E-9)	3.827E-11 (3.833E-9)
	2	7.275E-11 (7.291E-9)	4.850E-11 (4.861E-9)	5.416E-11 (5.427E-9)	5.323E-11 (5.334E-9)	6.315E-11 (6.328E-9)	8.731E-11 (8.758E-9)	8.520E-11 (8.537E-9)
	3	3.905E-11 (3.914E-9)	4.425E-11 (4.434E-9)	4.142E-11 (4.150E-9)	3.858E-11 (3.866E-9)	3.968E-11 (3.977E-9)	6.074E-11 (6.091E-9)	6.189E-11 (6.202E-9)
	4	6.866E-11 (6.880E-9)	6.284E-11 (6.297E-9)	6.567E-11 (6.581E-9)	5.361E-11 (5.381E-9)	4.630E-11 (4.640E-9)	4.992E-4 (5.003E-9)	3.858E-11 (3.866E-9)
	5	4.866E-11 (4.876E-9)	3.402E-11 (3.409E-9)	1.843E-11 (1.846E-9)	1.465E-11 (1.468E-9)	1.559E-11 (1.562E-9)	3.339E-11 (3.346E-9)	5.512E-11 (5.523E-9)
	6	3.858E-11 (3.866E-9)	3.197E-11 (3.2O4E-9)	4.992E-11 (5.003E-9)	9.921E-11 (9.942E-9)	6.535E-11 (6.549E-9)	4.693E-11 (4.703E-9)	5.717E-11 (5.224E-9)
	7	6.551E-11 (6.565E-9)	6.551E-11 (6.565E-9)	3.779E-11 (3.787E-9)	2.236E-11 (2.241E-9)	3.228E-11 (3.235E-9)	3.181E-11 (3.188E-9)	5.921E-11 (4.924E-9)
	8	4.598E-11 (4.608E-9)	4.283E-11 (4.292E-9)	4.992E-11 (5.601E-9)	4.614E-11 (4.628E-9)	4.898E-11 (4.908E-9)	3.622E-11 (3.630E-9)	———

(Values in parenthesis are dose exposure through dermal contact).

Table 3. Shows the hazard quotient of lead contacted through inhalation and dermal contact with scrapped car paint dust

S/N	Workshop	Vehicle 1	Vehicle 2	Vehicle 3	Vehicle 4	Vehicle 5	Vehicle 6	Vehicle 7
	1	1.498E-8 (1.501E-6)	1.818E-8 (1.822E-6)	1.687E-8 (1.691E-6)	1.521E-8 (1.524E-6)	9.539E-9 (9.559E-7)	9.763E-9 (9.784E-7)	1.093E-8 (1.096E-6)
	2	2.079E-8 (2.083E-6)	1.386E-8 (1.389E-6)	1.548E-8 (1.551E-6)	1.521E-8 (1.524E-6)	1.804E-8 (1.808E-6)	2.495E-8 (2.502E-6)	2.434E-8 (2.439E-6)
	3	1.116E-8 (1.115E-6)	1.264E-8 (1.267E-6)	1.183E-8 (1.186E-6)	1.102E-8 (1.105E-6)	1.134E-8 (1.136E-6)	1.093E-8 (1.096E-6)	1.764E-8 (1.768E-6)
	4	1.962E-8 (1.966E-6)	1.795E-8 (1.799E-6)	1.876E-8 (1.880E-6)	1.532E-8 (1.538E-6)	1,323E-8 (1.326E-6)	1.426E-8 (1.429E-6)	1.102E-8 (1.105E-6)
	5	1.390E-8 (1.393E-6)	9.719E-9 (9.739E-7)	5.264E-9 (5.275E-7)	4.184E-9 (4.464E-7)	4.454E-9 (4.464E-7)	9.539E-9 (9.559E-7)	1.575E-8 (1.578E-6)
	6	1.102E-8 (1.105E-6)	9.314E-9 (9.153E-7)	1.425E-8 (1.429E-6)	2.835E-8 (2.841E-5)	1.867E-8 (1.871E-6)	1.341E-8 (1.344E-6)	1.634E-8 (1.637E-6)
	7	1.872E-8 (1.876E-6)	1.872E-8 (1.876E-6)	1.080E-8 (1.876E-7)	6.389E-9 (6.403E-7)	9.224E-9 (9.243E-7)	9.089E-9 (9.108E-7)	1.692E-8 (1.695E-6)
	8	1.426E-8 (1.429E-6)	1.318E-8 (1.320E-6)	1.399E-8 (1.320E-6)	1.399E-8 (1.402E-6)	1.035E-8 (1.037E-6)	1.316E-8 (1.317E-6)	1.224E-8 (1.226E-6)

(Values in parenthesis are hazard quotient of dermal contact).

Table 4. Shows chronic hazard index of lead exposures contacted through inhalation and dermal contact with scrapped car paint dust

S/N	Workshop	Total No of Vehicle Per Workshop	Lead Exposure Route	
			Through Inhalation	Through Dermal Contact
	1	7	1.343E-8	1.346E-6
	2	7	1.895E-8	1900E-6
	3	7	1.16E-5	1.162E-6
	4	7	1.574E-8	1.577E-6
	5	7	8.97E-9	9.031E-7
	6	7	1.581E-9	1.584E-6
	7	7	1.284E-8	1.286E-6
	8	6	1.295E-8	1.297E-6

Table 2 shows the calculated dose exposure expressed in terms of a daily dose lead and for each exposure pathway. Specifically the doses contacted through inhalation of paint dust particles and the dose absorbed through the skin were presented in Table 2. Table 3 shows the hazard quotient of lead contacted through both inhalation and dermal contact. The exposure through dermal contact has a high risk values than exposure through inhalation. But the risk of all the vehicles in all the workshops were in the range of $X \times 10^{-8} - X \times 10^{-9}$ for exposure through inhalation while that of dermal contact is in the range of $X \times 10^{-6}$ to $X \times 10^{-7}$.

Table 4 shows the total hazard index of both inhalation and dermal exposure pathway. The HI for inhalation is in the range of 10^{-5} to 10^{-9} while that of dermal contact is $X \times 10^{-6}$ to $X \times 10^{-5}$, both are below one (1) showing that non-carcinogenic risk will not occur but that of workshop 3 with $X \times 10^{-5}$ through and all those of dermal contact are closer to one (1) and on continuous accumulation can lead to health risk.

Discussion

Scrapped car paint dust matrix contains an appreciable quantity of lead, with highest concentration values of 4.04 ± 0.09, 5.55 ± 0.03, 3.17 ± 0.00, 4.36 ± 0.04, 3.50 ± 0.01, 6.30 ± 0.01, 4.16 ± 0.01 and 3.17 ± 0.00 for vehicles 2, 6, 6, 1, 7, 4, 1, 2 and 3 for workshops 1-8 (Table 1), they can be considered high for a developing country like Nigeria without adequate technology for sustainable environmental remediation and public health care provision. High volume of importation of fairly used vehicle in Nigeria reputed to be the highest in Africa predisposes the country to heavy metal pollution. The desire of their owners to make do with what they have entails reworking of the automobiles – old car paints are scrapped, some parts are removed or panel-beat into proper shapes and re-welded before finishing and repainting.

Automobile accidents, another area Nigeria has "comparative advantage" because of questionable road worthiness of the imported automobiles have given rise to rickety vehicles dotting the Nigerian environment. Depending on the degree and severity of the accidents, some vehicles are irreparable while some are reworked, going through these processes of panel beating, welding, old paint scrapping and repainting. In some cases, where the vehicles can no longer be reworked because of the severity of the accident or in cases of natural breakdown of the vehicle due to natural expiration of the vehicular component, the rickety vehicle are left to the adverse effect of climate – high temperature and rainfall, leading to expansion, contraction and corrosion and consequent break down of components of the vehicle. The net effect is that high volume of heavy metals including lead (Pb) are continuously released into the Nigerian environment. The fact that the country lacks appropriate technology to deal with automobile waste coupled with no legislation on life span of vehicles that should be imported into Nigeria or that can ply Nigerian roads. Where legislation exists, its weak implementation or non compliance with standards makes the Nigerian environment especially soil and water a great reservoir of lead. A critical look at Table 1 shows that the lead levels are in an amount that can cause serious health problem when ingested, inhaled (equation 1) or when exposed to through dermal contact (equation 2). Lead (Pb) stands out as the most ubiquitous metal in Nigerian environment, caused by automobile emissions (Kakulu, 2003). Preliminary studies showed that lead air emissions at ground level in Lagos (Nigeria) are far higher than levels in the cities like London and New York, but similar to those of brazil or the Caribbean, due to perturbation by road side traffic (Fakayaode and Olu-Owolabi, 2003b). Exposure to lead expressed in terms of daily dose and calculated separately for each exposure pathway (inhalation and dermal contact, equation 1 and 2) using exposure point concentration (Table 1) was tabulated in Table 2. In comparison for all the workshops and vehicles examined, an individual working in automobile repair workshop or the general populace since the workshops are all located within residential areas, has the highest exposure risk to lead poisoning through dermal contact (equation 2, Table 2) than through inhalation (equation 1, Table 2), using the same exposure point concentration (Table 1). The doses of lead thus calculated for each vehicle in any given workshop and exposure pathway are subsequently divided by the reference dose of lead to yield a hazard quotient (HQ) or non-cancer risk (equation 3). Although lead presents a non-cancer risk value, it presents a toxicological profile, a chemical form that may occur in scrapped car paint dust matrix. The results of risk assessment using equation 3 are shown in Table 3, shows that dermal contact with scrapped car paint dust matrix is the route of exposure that results in a higher risk for lead, this agrees with the work of Ferreira – Baptista and De-Miguel (2005).

The chronic hazard index (HI) calculated from equation 4 and presented in Table 4 is the sum of more than one hazard quotient for multiple substances or multiple exposure pathways. In this study since we are considering only lead, the hazard index (HI) is the sum total of all the hazard quotient of all the seven (7) vehicles in all the workshops except workshop eight (8) with six (6) vehicles, presented separately for each exposure pathway (inhalation and dermal contact, Table 4). Where HI values >1, shows that there is a chance that non-carcinogenic risk may occur and when HI <1, the reverse applies (Liu et al., 2013). The result in Table 4 of this study shows that HI<1 applies for both exposure pathway, but exposure through dermal contact is closer to HI>1 and on continuous exposure could be detrimental to health. The risks of all vehicles in all the workshops where in the range of $X \times 10^{-8}$ to $X \times 10^{-9}$ for exposure through inhalation while that of dermal contact is in the range of $X \times 10^{-6}$ to $X \times 10^{-7}$ (Table 3). This hazard index (HI) for inhalation is in the range of $X \times 10^{-5}$ to $X \times 10^{-9}$ while that of dermal contact is $X \times 10^{-6}$ to $X \times 10^{-7}$ but that of workshop 3 with $X \times 10^{-5}$ through inhalation and that of dermal contact are closer to one (Table 4). This implies that the total non-carcinogenic hazard indices for both inhalation and dermal contact fell below the hazard threshold value of one (1) set by the U.S. EPA (U.S. EPA, 2011). This implies that the chance of non-cancer risk resulting from a day exposure through either inhalation or dermal contact is unlikely; however, heavy metals are cumulative due to their long half-lives and their build up overtime could be detrimental. This work amongst numerous others (Orisakwe et al., 1996; Orisakwe et al., 2004; Nduka et al., 2008) is an indication that occupational and direct local exposure (Ma et al., 2008) is the most self-evident scenario of lead or chemicals associated with electronic/automobile.

Exposure Scenario

In this present work, we considered only two exposure pathway (inhalation and dermal contact), but suffice it to say that humans could be exposed to lead poisoning via six main pathways: (1) direct ingestion of lead contaminated soil particles (2) dermal contact with soil/paint dust (3) direct through the food chain (4) inhalation of soil/paint dust from the air (5) oral intake from ground water and (6) dermal intake from ground water. So many activities may involve exposures through the above routes. The main routes of exposure for Pb^{2+} are inhalation and ingestion. Inhalation exposure to Pb^{2+} is a much more efficient route of absorption than ingestion, with an estimated absorption efficiency ratio of 10:1 in the lung compared to the gastrointestinal tract (Wells et al., 1975). Absorption of Pb^{2+} from the intestine is mediated by both passive and facilitated diffusion, although passive diffusion plays a minor role in total absorption (Angust and Fung, 1981). Several studies on the intestinal absorption of Pb^{2+} have shown evidence of carrier mediated transport but the identity of the transporter(s) is still a matter of debate (Barton et al., 1978; Fullmer, 1990). Lead can be absorbed through the skin (Sun et al., 2002; Filon et al., 2006), although studies on the dermal absorption of lead in humans are still scarce, damaged skin, pH and metallic chemical structure are likely factors that could enhance percutaneous penetration of metals (Filon et al., 2009; Hostynek, 2003).

Occupational Exposure

In our previous work (Nduka et al, 2008b), in which urine samples of occupational exposed artisans in Awka South Eastern Nigeria were analysed for lead, the results showed urine samples of auto-mechanics with an average lead concentration of 0.07mg/L, "Okada" (motorcycle) riders (0.05mg/L), filling station (fuel) attendants (0.04mg/L) while students who served as control had an average urine lead concentration of 0.01mg/L. It is a fact that lead toxicity could occur through several other sources, but the very small average lead levels of 0.01mg/L of the control (student) confirms that the source of contamination may be leaded petrol whose exposure pathway is inhalation. Although the right sample to use for the study would have been blood but for the difficulty in collecting blood samples because of cultural and religious suspicious belief. The presence of lead in urine, an excretory product is an indication of higher lead levels in blood (Nduka et al., 2008b). Inhalation of fugitive dust particles can predispose an individual to lead poisoning. Analysis of soil dust particles in seven (7) municipal cities of South Eastern Nigeria (Aba, Awka, Enugu, Onitsha, Nnewi, Warri and Port-Harcourt) showed an average concentration in the range of 0.10 – 0.48mg/kg of dust. (Nduka and Orisakwe, 2010), this is far above US EPA MCL of 0.015mg/L of lead in drinking water.

Even though one can be exposed to lead through paint dust matrix and soil dust through dermal contact, the surest means of dermal contact is through cosmetics, in a comparative health risk assessment of locally and imported cosmetics in Nigeria, the result showed that 42.86% of the locally made cosmetics had average lead values in the range of 0.13 – 1.32mg/kg whereas those imported had various lead levels ranging from 0.1 – 42.12mg/kg (Nduka et al., 2015). The most versatile exposure pathway is through ingestion because exposure through dermal contact as with case of cosmetics may be a matter of choice but exposure through ingestion or inhalation may not be, nutrition and inhalation are normal physiological activities. Herbal remedies and preparations are a significant route of exposure through ingestion, as over 80% of the populations in some Asian and African countries depend on traditional medicine for primary health care (WHO, 2008). Globally, especially in developing countries, survey has proved that 75-80% of the population patronize herbal medications (Kamboj, 2000; Crawford et al., 2006). In one of the recent study of heavy metals in Nigerian herbal remedies, it was shown that 54.17% of the samples (all solids) violated both the WHO and EU safe limits for lead with percentage violation in the range of 16 – 106% (Igweze et al., 2012). Alongside with herbal remedy in exposure to lead through ingestion (nutrition) is kitchen utensils and water. Imported glazed ceramics (drinking mugs, soup bowls and cooking pots) has been reported to contain more lead than those that were locally manufactured (Ketiku and Adeyinka, 1999) while sachet water which was before now thought to be the safest form of drinking water in Nigeria, was later discovered to be a subtle means of heavy metal exposure including lead (Orisakwe et al., 2006). Contamination of foods by heavy metals has become an inevitable challenge these days. Flooding from heavy down pour may lead to horizontal leaching from dump sites causing metal uptake by root of crops; plant uptake is one of the major pathways by which heavy metals in soils enter the human food chain. Plant shoots have been found to be contaminated by heavy metals.

In case of children, maternal dietary habits influence risk of heavy metal exposure to infants. Lead is present in breast milk as an indication of levels found in maternal blood supplied to the fetus during gestation (Dorea, 2004). The work of Manton et al., (2003), shows that blood lead levels of nursing mothers continue to rise reaching a maximum of 6 – 8 months after delivery, but pregnancy to pregnancy blood lead levels falls implying that the greatest risk of lead toxicity lies with first pregnancy.

Another major route of exposure to lead in Nigeria is commonly administered pediatric syrup (Orisakwe and Nduka, 2009). It is common practice for doctors to recommend drugs known to cure specific ailments (such as indigestion, headache, malaria, cough, measles, cold, catarrh, anaemia, stomach upset etc) to pregnant women and lactating mothers and children. The lead levels in our pediatric syrup compared well with those of canned and non-canned beverages (Maduabuchi et al., 2006) and that of sachet water (Orisakwe et al., 2006). A possible route of lead into these drugs may be during processing such as lead solder, use of contaminated water, poor assaying of raw materials, packaging, poor hygiene and storage facilities.

Consumption of pediatric syrup is a regular affair in Nigeria because most of them are over the counter drugs, frequent health problem coupled with weak health institutions which are hallmark of underdevelopment, weak and struggling economy, lack of political will, poverty and weak leadership predisposes the populace to self help. The literacy level is also a contributing factor as large population still indulges in self medication. In a prevalence study of parental medication on children before going to hospital performed by Orisakwe et al., (1994), 99% of children aged 1 – 6years were found to have received it before seeing a doctor. About 39% of the studied population had taken at least two drugs before been taken to the hospital. The most frequently administered drugs were paracetamol and chloroquine. In a rural setting, such that abound in Nigeria, where the only potable water supply are streams, ditches, ponds, rivulets, lakes, rivers etc (surface water) which are wide open to various contaminants such as lead. These surface water including occasionally dug and underground water is the only source of water for drinking, laundry, cooking and other domestic needs (Nduka and Orisakwe, 2009; Nduka and Orisakwe, 2007). The implication is that the general population strata are exposed to lead poisoning and other chemical species. These environmental pollutants which are environmentally mobile tend to accumulate in organisms and become persistent because of their chemical stability or poor biodegradability (Emoyan et al., 2005), therefore consumption of marine foods such as crayfish, crabs, periwinkle, fish etc, which is a daily delicacy especially in the river-rine communities of Nigeria, is a veritable means of lead exposure. We have established that different marine fish species in the Niger Delta region of Nigeria with its attendant crude oil and fractional spillages are laden with heavy metals including lead (Nduka et al., 2010; Nduka et al., 2006).

Comparative Study

Major adult exposure to lead include food which is believed to account for over 60% of blood lead levels, air inhalation accounts for nearly 30% while water is of 10% (John et al., 1991). Concentration exposures to lead in this study can be compared with others, limiting comparison to few of our studies. Although it has be stated that primary means of exposure to lead is through drinking water from lead-based plumbing materials (US EPA, 1989), but exposure point concentration in water cannot be as much as through industrial activities like mining, smelting, refining and manufacturing processes, ingestion of lead in flaking lead paints in old houses, in lead-containing objects and in contaminated food (Bruening et al., 1999), cosmetics, soil, infant formulae, road surface wear, particulate emissions and lubricating oil (Zhou et al., 2007; Pruvot et al., 2006, Duzgoren-Aydin, 2007).

Refuse dump soils, flaked paints from building and road side surface soils (Tables 5, 6 and 7) are high in lead concentration when contrasted with the results of our study (Table 1). An individual may be exposed to lead poisoning through ingestion of soil and flaked paints (Tables 5, 6 and 7), this may not be a problem for adult but a risk for children and yet may be an occasional issue even for adults, this present study is occupational exposure and therefore with high severity risk.

Table 5. Concentration of Lead (Pb) at refuse dumpsites in Awka. South-eastern Nigeria

S/N	Site	Depth (m)	Lead (Pb) Level
	Site A	0.00 1.35	350 (83.8) 510
	Site B	0.00 1.35	500 (ND) 350
	Site C	0.00 1.35	620 (ND) 613.50
	Site D	0.00 1.35	401 (3.80) 370
	Site E	0.00 1.35	145.30 (ND) 160.30

(Nd: Not detected, Control values in parenthesis, Nduka et al., 2008).

Table 6. Lead levels in flaked paints from buildings of South-eastern Nigeria

S/No	City	Age of Building	Use of Building	Lead Levels (mg/kg)
	Enugu	0 – 5 years 6 – 10 years 11years and above	Residential Commercial Residential	69.843 ± 4.886 39.385 ± 1.111 43.005 ± 0.077
	Onitsha	0 – 5 years 6 – 10 years 11years and above	Residential Commercial Residential	60.013 ± 0.000 74.352 ± 0.571 49.503 ± 0.000
	Aba	0 – 5 years 6 – 10 years 11years and above	Residential Commercial Residential	54.627 ± 0.000 66.432 ± 0.013 42.567 ± 0.003
	Port-Harcourt	0 – 5 years 6 – 10 years 11years and above	Residential Commercial Residential	66.718 ± 0.001 58.682 ± 0.001 51.806 ± 0.285

(Nduka et al., 2008).

Table 7. Lead levels of roadside surface soil in cities of South-eastern Nigeria

S/N	Year	Town	Road One		Road Two	
			Point One	Point Two	Point One	Point Two
	2007	Enugu	10.29 ± 0.01 (0.88)	28.20 ± 0.00 (1.64)	27.12 ± 0.01 (1.20)	17.06 ± 0.01 (0.92)
	2007	Awka	6.47 ± 0.02 (0.44)	6.31 ± 0.02 (0.21)	14.11 ± 0.00 (0.48)	14.16 ± 0.11 (0.78)
	2007	Nnewi	33.40 v 0.01 (1.66)	13.92 ± 0.00 (0.75)	24.35 ± 0.00 (0.66)	10.29 ± 0.00 (0.28)
	2007	Aba	16.64 ± 0.25 (0.78)	17.77 ± 0.07 (1.32)	22.56 ± 0.01 (2.12)	17.36 ± 0.02 (1.02)
	2007	Onitsha	20.00 ± 0.00 (4.22)	38.99 ± 0.01 (2.10)	19.60 ± 0.00 (0.87)	14.78 ± 0.00 (0.48)
	2007	Port-Harcourt	7.43 ± 0.00 (0.24)	12.82 ± 0.00 (0.36)	13.08 ± 0.01 (0.56)	9.23 ± 0.01 (0.38)
	2007	Warri	8.00 ± 0.00 (0.08)	4.75 ± 0.00 (0.02)	4.75 ± 0.00 (0.04)	8.75 ± 0.00 (0.06)
	2008	Enugu	14.50 ± 0.01 (2.85)	12.06 ± 0.01 (1.06)	10.00 ± 0.01 (0.78)	11.96 ± 0.01 (1.12)
	2008	Awka	18.82 ± 0.00 (1.96)	18.14 ± 0.01 (0.76)	16.47 ± 0.02 (1.89)	15.96 ± 0.01 (0.64)
	2008	Nnewi	44.09 ± 0.00 (1.12)	82.28 ± 0.01(3.21)	119.20 ± 0.00 (4.67)	4,238.29 ± 0.00 (8.44)
	2008	Aba	16.41 ± 0.01 (0.98)	13.08 ± 0.01 (1.53)	21.28 ± 0.00 (0.44)	17.18 ± 0.01 (1.32)
	2008	Onitsha	16.13 ± 0.01 (1.32)	10.96 ± 0.00 (0.42)	10.97 ± 0.01 (0.22)	80.36 ± 0.00 (1.42)
	2008	Port-Harcourt	30.51 ± 0.02 (5.87)	21.28 ± 0.01 (0.36)	89.75 ± 0.03 (1.32)	12.31 ± 0.01 (0.12)
	2008	Warri	7.75 ± 0.67 (0.82)	5.00 ± 0.00 (0.12)	8.75 ± 0.00 (0.24)	6.00 ± 0.00 (0.07)

(N = 3, Control values in parenthesis, Nduka and Orisakwe, 2010).

Table 8. Shows lead levels (mg/L) of pediatric syrups

S/N	Pharmaceutical Product	Batch No	NAFDAC No	MFG Date	Expiry Date	Metal Level (mg/L) of Pb	Place of Manufacture
	Bellis Cough Syrup	9601	04 – 1814	June 2006	June 2009	Nd	Southport, England
	MIM Iron Syrup	003705xP	04 – 5942	June 2007	May 2010	Nd	Mumbai, India
	Pentax Paracetamol Syrup	L41006	04 – 0073	Oct. 2006	Sept. 2008	Nd	Lagos, Nigeria (Licensed by Vitabiotics, England)
	Woodwards Gripe Water	070048	04 – 1030	Aug. 2007	Aug. 2010	Nd	Lagos, Nigeria (Licensed by Woodward, England)
	Menthodex Cough Syrup	672H1	04 – 0971	June 2007	June 2010	Nd	United Kingdom
	Chloramphenicol	71002	04 – 2745	Oct. 2007	Oct. 2010	Nd	Sango-Ota, Nigeria (licensed by Omega Mayor, Jersey)
	Erythromycin Suspension	007	04 – 5863	Nov. 2005	Nov. 2008	Nd	Buchistan, Pakistan
	Cephalexin Syrup	061624A	04 – 0883	Jan. 2006	Jan. 2009	Nd	Cairo, A.R.E., Egypt
	Vardorange Syrup	VO – 21	04 – 6063	Feb. 2006	Jan. 2009	0.02	Mumbai, India
	Ailon Multivitamin Drop	360345	04 – 3204	Nov. 2006	Oct. 2008	0.03	London SEI 751, England
	Haemoglobin Syrup	37527	04 – 7608	Feb. 2006	Jan. 2010	Nd	Tipperart, Ireland
	Halfan	6005	04 – 2181	March 2006	March 2009	Nd	Nanterre, France
	Zentel Albendazole	370001	04 – 2467	Jan. 2007	Dec. 2009	0.03	Bangalore, India
	Maxiquine	L8107	04 – 5253	Jan. 2007	Dec. 2009	0.09	Lagos, Nigeria (Licensed by Vitabiotic, England)
	Piccan	5724	04 – 2729	July 2007	July 2010	Nd	Dublin, Ireland
	Cadiphen	E7015	04 – 1876	May 2007	April 2011	0.01	Dholka, India
	Asco-J Vitamin	0020	04 – 7233	Aug. 2007	Aug. 2009	0.03	Enugu, Nigeria
	Emvite	4110K	04 – 0135	Aug. 2007	Aug. 2010	0.41	Lagos, Nigeria
	J-Vite	0018	04 – 7232	July 2007	July 2009	0.14	Enugu, Nigeria
	Ferobin Plus	LA79138	04 – 4838	June 2007	May 2010	0.09	Ogun, Nigeria

Table 8. (Continued)

S/N	Pharmaceutical Product	Batch No	NAFDAC No	MFG Date	Expiry Date	Metal Level (mg/L) of Pb	Place of Manufacture
	Emzolyn	3050K	04 – 1454	May 2007	May 2010	0.17	Lagos, Nigeria
	Multivite	71434012	04 – 0031	June 2007	Nov. 2008	0.05	Ogun, Nigeria
	Kingsize Vit C	HM2279C	04 – 0879	Jan. 2006	Dec. 2008	0.10	Ogidi, Nigeria
	Asco J Vit. C	0020	04 – 7233	Aug. 2007	Aug. 2009	0.02	Enugu, Nigeria
	Guaze Vit. C	G200152	04 – 3174	Feb. 2007	Feb. 2009	Nd	Awka, Nigeria
	Em-Vit C	807K	04 – 0262	Feb. 2007	Feb. 2009	Nd	Lagos, Nigeria
	Zvobes Cough Syrup	007	04 – 0665	Feb. 2006	Feb. 2009	Nd	Lagos, Nigeria
	Gauze Multivitamin	00213	04 – 3234	Feb. 2007	Feb. 2009	Nd	Awka, Nigeria
	Gaviron	GVM – 0049	04 – 5131	Feb. 2007	Feb. 2010	0.20	Awka, Nigeria
	Coflin	11907	04 – 0540	Sept. 2007	August 2009	Nd	Lagos, Nigeria
	Avipol	ASV02	04 – 4744	June 2007	May 2010	Nd	Ogun, Nigeria
	Cypri Gold	260807	04 – 1627	Aug. 2007	July 2009	Nd	Lagos, Nigeria
	Haemoglobin Tonic	001HV	04 – 0338	July 2007	July 2010	0.12	Lagos, Nigeria
	Emzoron Tonic	4327K	04 – 1450	July 2007	July 2009	0.15	Lagos, Nigeria
	Babyrex	T8881	04 – 3937	Nov. 2007	Oct. 2010	Nd	Ilorin, Nigeria
	Gauze Chloroquine	TN00151	04 – 3166	Jan. 2006	Feb. 2009	0.001	Awka, Nigeria
	Septrin Syrup	6002	04 – 1888	Oct. 2006	Oct. 2009	0.02	Ogun, Nigeria
	KP Multivitamin Syrup	HM2199M	NA	Feb. 2007	Jan. 2009	0.96	Ogidi, Nigeria
	Seven Keys Herbal Mixture	1791008	04 – 1986L	Oct. 2007	Oct. 2010	0.12	Onitsha, Nigeria
	Phenergan	LOTTW1200	04 – 0290	June 2006	August 2009	0.08	Lagos, Nigeria
	Magcid Suspension	MD0065	04 – 5136	Nov. 2007	Nov. 2009	1.08	Awka, Nigeria

S/N	Pharmaceutical Product	Batch No	NAFDAC No	MFG Date	Expiry Date	Metal Level (mg/L) of Pb	Place of Manufacture
	Jawaron Syrup	L7019	04 – 2037	July 2007	June 2009	Nd	Lagos, Nigeria
	Diastop Suspension	7011	04 – 1393	Jan. 2007	Jan. 2011	0.04	Lagos, Nigeria
	Piriton Syrup	7K5 4008	04 – 0437	Oct. 2007	Sept. 2010	0.02	Ogun, Nigeria
	2.2.1 Forte Chloroquine Sulphate	LOTIX -120	04 – 1718	Jan. 2007	Dec. 2010	Nd	Lagos Nigeria
	Paracetamol Syrup	1124M	04 – 0289	Jan. 2008	Jan. 2011	Nd	Lagos, Nigeria
	Tixylix Cough Syrup	TW815	04 – 0320	Sept. 2006	August 2009	0.09	Lagos, Nigeria
	Broncholyte	BI 63	04 – 2904	Dec. 2007	Dec. 2010	Nd	Ogun, Nigeria
	Colipan	B 109	04 – 4044	August 2007	August 2010	Nd	Ogun, Nigeria
	Em-B-Plex	3487K	04 – 0287	July 2007	July 2010	Nd	Lagos, Nigeria

(Orisakwe and Nduka., 2009).

This is because an artisan engaged in vehicle panel beating – welding, scrapping and repainting (re-working) of vehicles is a lifelong exposure. The cumulative effect may be life threatening. One of the most prevalent and neglected diseases in Nigeria and most of the sub-Saharan African countries probably is lead poisoning which has affected a large fraction of the childhood population because of the growing multiplicity of potential exposure routes, yet the diagnostic rate of ailments associated with lead poisoning by Nigerian medical personnel is scanty. This point is amplified by the fact that only three studies of childhood lead poisoning with limited sample sizes have been conducted in Nigeria (Nriagu et al., 1996; Pfitzner et al., 2000; Wright et al., 2005). In a recent update in Nigeria by Orisakwe (2009), the high blood lead levels (BLL) have documented not only in occupational cohorts but also in "unexposed" control subjects. The high BLL among controls cast doubts as how unexposed are these 'unexposed control subject' actually are. Given the high volume of consumption of packaged waters, canned and un-canned beverages in apparent attempt of Nigerians to adopt a western lifestyle, coupled with effect of climate change – high perspiration due to high temperature especially during the dry season, the question arises of the long term effect of waters and beverages with various levels of lead on human health. The concentration of lead in sachet water (Table not shown), that of pediatric syrup (Table 8) and canned/un-canned beverages (Table not shown) where they were detectable, are nearly equal in concentration. In a study by Orisakwe and co-workers (2006), in which it was shown that 12.2% of the sachet water samples studied had lead levels exceeding the EPA MCL of 0.015mg/L are thought provoking. These findings are of great concern because of the increased epidemiologic and experimental evidence of the adverse health effect of lead even at lower levels (Davis et al., 1993). The level of lead in drinking water is of prime concern because plumbism (chronic lead poisoning) has also been associated with reduced gestational age and birth weight, as well as hypertension, lower heamaglobin levels and impairment of renal function, among other effects (NRC, 1993; Vupputuri et al., 2003). Most lead values of pediatric syrup and canned/un-canned beverages also exceeded the US EPA MCL of 0.015mg/L of lead for drinking water (Tables 8 and 9). Although the concentration of lead in our present study (Table 1), is very high in comparison with that of sachet water (Tables not shown), pediatric syrups (Table 8) and that of canned/un-canned beverages (Table not shown), the exposure through these three (sachet water, pediatric syrup and canned/un-canned beverages) are ubiquities. The general population consumes them even in large volume all year round. Some of the syrups are for general ailments such as malaria, so no age limit in usage. An individual engaged in automobile vehicle re-working in addition to its exposure (occupational) will also engage in drinking sachet water, syrups and canned/un-canned beverages.

Health Implications of Lead Exposure

Exposure to lead has serious health implication as all ages are at risk. Lead is a neurotoxin responsible for most common type of human metal toxicosis (Beman, 1980). Low-level lead exposure has been associated with reduced IQ (Needleman, 1993) and with attention deficit disorders in children (Yule and Rutter, 1985). Lead poisoning is the 6th most important contributor to global burden of diseases measure in disability adjusted life years (DALYS), with sub-Saharan African countries being predominantly responsible for the global DALYS (Pruss-Ustun and Corvalan, 2006). A study in Nigeria found elevated blood lead levels in a large proportion of Nigerian children, it was shown that one quarter of the children tested in Nigeria had blood lead levels (BLL) over 10μg/dL and the value for about 4% of the children exceeded 20μg/dL (Nriagu et al., 2008). This compared well with that of China where the mean concentration of lead in the blood of children living in Guiyu, China, a notorious destination for improper e-waste recycling (Stone, 2009) is 15μg/dL.

There is no known safe level of exposure to lead; remedial action is recommended for children with levels above 10μg/dL (Huo et al., 2007). This is because children run the greatest risk of lead poisoning in inner city areas of Nigeria where inhalation and ingestion of metals like lead and cadmium from dust and ashes are common (Fakayode and Olu-Owolabi, 2003). Hyperactivity, anorexia, decreased play activity; low intelligence quotient and poor school performance have been observed in children with high lead levels (Needleman and Bellinger, 1991). Children are more susceptible to the effects of the lead than adults for a number of reasons: (1) Children with hand to mouth behavior are at particular risk of elevated lead exposure due to the ingestion of lead dust (Gibson, 2005). (2) Another factor is that children have a higher intake of lead than adults. Adult human absorption of lead is around 10% (Hursh and Suomela, 1968), while infant's absorption of lead is about 26.2% (Ziegler et al., 1978). Partly due to increased absorption, children have a higher burden of mobile Pb^{2+} stores, because they store less lead in bone, it results in a higher BPb burden (Neal and Guilarte, 2012). Lead crosses the placenta during pregnancy and has been associated with intrauterine death, prematurity and low birth weight. Adult exposures occurs more frequently at the work place and primarily involves the central nervous system, symptoms of hemoepotic system involvement include microcytic, hypochromic anemia with basophilic stippling of the erythrocytes (Emory et al., 1999). Although blood lead leavel BLL < 10mg/dL is currently considered as the threshold for concern in the United States (CDC, 2007), several studies has shown that there is no safe dose for lead exposure especially among children (Rogan and Ware, 2003). Blood lead levels below 10mg/dL have been associated with impaired neuro-psychosocial development, delayed physical development and small stature, delayed onset of menarche and auditory problems (Min et al., 2008). Lead poisoning is also capable of inhibiting the final step in heme synthesis by interfering with the activity of the enzymes δ-aminolevulinic dehydratase (ALAD) and ferrochelatase leading to ZPP accumulation (Counter et al., 2007; Soldina et al., 2003). Lead because of its size and charge similarity, can substitute for calcium and included in bone. About 94% of the human Pb^{2+} body burden is found in bone in adults but only 73% in children. Pb^{2+} readily displaces Ca^{2+} in the bone matrix by cation-exchange process (Pounds et al., 1991). Lead in bone is not harmful but if high levels of calcium are ingested, lead in bone is replaced, then free lead in the body system may cause nephrotoxicity, neutrotoxicity and hypertension. Children because of high calcium assimilation due to developing skeletal systems require high calcium levels (Osmond et al., 1995). Recycling of Pb^{2+} between bone and blood occurs continuously, if recycling between blood and bone compartments could be eliminated the half-life of Pb^{2+} in blood would drop from 40days to about 10days (Brito et al., 2005). In blood, Pb^{2+} is primarily bound to protein. Up to 40% of blood Pb^{2+} (BPb) is bound to serum albumin and the remaining BPb is bound to sulfhydryl – or thiol – containing ligands (Al-Modhefer et al., 1991). High intra-erythrocyte concentration of lead can also affect several essential cellular processes adversely, including inhibition of protein synthesis (Graziano et al., 1991). Lead has a high affinity for the side chains of many proteins such as transferring (Qian et al., 1997), mobilferrin (Conrad et al., 1990), divalent metal-ion transporter, DMT1 (Gunshin et al., 1997), hemoglobin (Barltrop and Smith, 1972), and enzymes of heme synthesis (Goldberg, 1972). The ability of Pb^{2+} to undergo metathesis reactions with Zn^{2+} and Ca^{2+} metalloproteins resulting in loss of metabolic function continues to be a primary hypothesis underlying the detrimental effects of lead exposure (Lewis and Cohen, 2004).

Metabolic balance studies showed that Pb^{2+} is predominantly excreted through feces, with urinary excretion playing a secondary role. Trace amounts of Pb^{2+} can also be excreted through hair, sweat, breast milk and nails (Pounds et al., 1978; Rabinowitz et al., 1974; Ziegler et al., 1978).

Lead poisoning can moderate the susceptibility of a child to many parasitic diseases, including infections from vector-borne, food-borne, water-borne or soil transmitted pathogens thereby increasing the disease burden in the community. But lead may be helpful anyways, recently, studies confirm that lead protects against parasitemia in individuals (Nriagu et al., 2008) as well as in plasmodium-infected mice (Kempe et al., 2005; Koka et al., 2007). It has been established that low levels of lead in women of childbearing age can have adverse effect on their reproductive health and/or offspring (Bellinger, 2005). Lead has also been linked to infertility and miscarriage. Mendola et al., (2008) examined published studies and research reports from 1999 to 2007 indexed in PubMed and found that exposure to lead is the strongest environmental contaminant that interferes with healthy reproductive function in adult females.

Conclusion

There is no question that lead is a toxic heavy metal whose exposure route keeps increasing. We are not aware of any work on lead level of automobile scrapped paint dusts. The results of the present study shows that an artisan working in numerous automobile re-working workshops in Nigeria, may be accumulating higher doses of lead on daily bases. The results of already published articles indicate that children, pregnant women, nursing mothers and including artisans (such as auto-mechanics, painters, filling station fuel attendants, welders, and miners) are more at risk. Heavy metals including lead exposures may in part be responsible for increasing cases of non communicable ailments in Nigeria.

References

Agency for Toxic Substances and Diseases Registry (ATSDRY, 1992). Case studies in environmental medicine – lead toxicity. US Department of Health and Human Services: Washington, DC, USA.

Al-Modhefer AJ, Bradbury MW, Simons TJ (1991). Observations on the chemical nature of lead in human blood serum. *Clin. Sci.* (London). 81: 823 – 829.

Angust BJ, Fung HL (1981). Kinetic characterisation of in vitro lead transport across the rat small intestine: Mechanism of intestinal lead transport. *Toxicol. Appl. Pharmacol.* 61: 39 – 47.

Anon (1996). Lead Pollution: A blight on the future. African Health; 18: 7.

Barltrop D, Smith A (1972). Lead binding to human haemoglobin. Experientia. 28: 76 – 77.

Barton JC, Contrad ME, Nuby S, Harrison L (1978). Effects of iron on the absorption and retention of lead. *J. Lab Clin Med.* 92: 536 – 547.

Bellinger DC (2005). "Teratogen update: Lead and pregnancy". *Birth Defects Research A*; 73 (6): 409 – 420.

Beman E (1980). Toxic metals and their analysis. Philadelphia: Hayden and Sons.

Brito JA, McNeil FE, Webber CE, Chettle DR (2005). Grid search: An innovative method for the estimation of the rates of lead exchange between body compartments. *J. Environ. Monit.* 7: 241 – 247.

Bruening K, Kemp FN, Simone N, Holding Y, Louria DB, Bogden JD (1999). Dietary calcium intakes of urban children at risk of lead poisoning. *Environ Health Perspect;* 107: 431 – 435.

Centres for Disease Control (CDC, 2007).Third national report on human exposure to environmental chemicals. Centres for the Disease Control. Atlanta.CA.www.cdc.gov/exposivereport/3rd/pdf/thirdreport.pdfs. (Assessed July, 2007)

Conrad ME, Umbreit JN, Moore EG (1991).A role for mucin in the absorption of inorganic iron and other metal cations. Astudy in rats. Gastroenterology. 100: 129 – 136.

Counter SA, Buchanan LH, Ortega F, Rifai N,Shannon MW (2007). Comparative analysis of zinc protoporphyrin and blood lead levels in lead-exposed Andean children. *Clin. Biochem.* 40:787 – 792.

Crawford NW, Cincotta DR, lim A, Powell CV (2006). A cross sectional survey of complementary and alternative medicine use by children and adolescents attending the university hospital of Wales; BMC *Complementary and Alternative Medicine;* 6: 16.

Davis JM, Elias RW, Grant LD (1993). Current issues in human lead exposures and regulation of lead. Neurotoxicol; 14: 15 – 27.

Dorea JG (2004). Mercury and lead during breastfeeding. *Br. J. Nutr*; 92 (1): 21 – 40.

Duzgoren – Aydin NS (2007).Sources and characteristics of lead pollution in the urban envirronment of Guangzhou. *Sci. Total. Envirron.*385: 182 – 195.

Emory E, Pattilo R, Archiobold E, Baryorn M, Sung F (1999). Neurobehavioral effects of low level lead exposure in human neonates. *AM. J. Obstet. Gynecol.* 181: 2 – 11.

Emoyan OO, Ogban FE, Akarah E (2005).Evaluation of heavy metals loading of river Ijana, Nigeria. *J. Appl. Sci. Environ. Manag.* 10 (2): 121 – 127.

Fakayode S, Olu-Owolabi I (2003). Trace metal content and estimated daily human intake from chicken eggs in Ibadan. Nigeria. *Arch. Environ. Health*; 58 (4): 245 – 251.

Fakayode SO, Olu-Owolabi BI(2003b). Heavy metal contamination of roadside topsoil in Osogbo, Nigeria: Its relationship to traffic density and proximity to highways. *Environ. Geol*; 44: 150 -157.

Ferreira-Baptista L, Demigul E (2005). Geochemistry and risk assessment of street dust in Luanda Angola: A Tropical Urban Environment. Atmospheric Environment 4 (71): DOI:01.1016/j.atmosenu.2005.03.026.

Filon FL, Boeniger M, Maino G, Adami G, Spinelli P, Damian A (2006). "Skin absorption of inorganic lead (PbO) and the effect of skin cleansers. *J. Occup. Environ. Med.* 48 (7): 692 – 699.

Filon FL, D'Agostin F, Crosera M, Adami G, Bovenzi M, Marina G (2009).In vitro absorption of metal powders through intact and damaged human skin. *Toxicology in Vitro*. 23 (4): 574 – 579.

Frazzoli C, Orisakwe OE, Dragone R, Mantovani A (2010). Diagnostic health risk assessment of electronic waste on the general population in developing countries scenarios.Environmental Impact Assessment Review. 30 (6): 388 – 399.

Fullmer CS (1990). International lead and calcium absorption: effect of 1, 25-dihydroxycholecalciferol and status. *Proc. Soc. Exp. Biol Med.* 194: 258 – 264.

Gibson JL (2005). A plea for painted railings and painted walls of rooms as the source of lead poisoning amongst Queensland children. 1904 Public *Health Rep.* 120: 301 – 304.

Goldberg A (1972). Lead poisoning and heme biosynthesis. *Br. J. Haematol.* 23: 521 – 524.

Graziano JH, Slavkovic V, Factor-Litvak P, Popovac D, Ahmedi X, Mehmeti A (1991). Depressed serum erythropoietin in pregnant women with elevated blood lead. *Arch. Environ. Health.* 46: 347 – 350.

Gunshin H, Mackenzie B, Berger UV, Gunshin Y, Romero MF, Boron WF, Nussberger S, Gollan JL, Hediger MA (1997). Cloning and characterization of a mammalian proton-coupled metal-ion transporter. *Nature*. 388: 482 – 488.

Hostynek JJ (2003). Factors determining percutaneous metal absorption. *Food and Chemical Toxicology*; 41 (3): 327 – 345.

Huo X, Peng L, Xu X, Zheng L, Qiu B, Qi Z, Zhang B, Han D, Piao Z (2007). Elevated blood lead levels of children in Guiyu, an electronic waste recycling town in China. *Environ. Health Perspect*. 115 (7): 1113 - 1117.

Hursh JB, Suomela J (1968). Absorption of 212Pb from the gastrointestinal tract of man. *Act. Radiol. Ther. Phys. Biol.* 7: 108 – 120.

Igweze ZN, Orisakwe OE, Obianime AW (2012). Nigerian herbal remedies and heavy metals: violation of standard recommended guidelines. *Asian Pacific Journal of Tropical Biomedicine*. 1 – 6.

John H, Cherly H, Richards S, Christine S (1991). Toxica A to Z, a guide to everyday pollution hazards. University of California Press; Berkeley, Los Angeles. Ca, USA/Oxford, UK. 47 – 104.

Kakulu SE (2003). Trace metal concentration in roadside surface soil and tree bark: A measurement of local atmospheric pollution in Abuja, Nigeria. *Environmental Monit Assess*; 89 (3): 233 – 242.

Kamboj VP (2000). Herbal medicine. Current Science. 78: 35 – 39.

Kempe DS, Lang PA, Eisele K, Klarl BA, Weider T, Huber SM, Duranton C, Lang F (2005). Stimulation of erythrocyte phosphatidylserine exposure by lead ions. *Am. J. Physiol. Cell. Physiol*. 288: C396 – C402.

Ketiku AD, Adeyinka O (1999). Leaching of lead from imported and Nigeria eathenware pottery and ceramic household utensils into food and drinks. *Biol. Appl. Chem.* 44: 18 – 20.

Koka S, Huber SM, Boini KM, Lang C, Foller M, Lang F (2007). Lead decreases parasitemia and enhances survival of plasmodium berghei-infected mice. *Biochem. Biophys. Res. Communic*. 363: 484 – 489.

Lee JD (1996). Concise inorganic chemistry. 5th Edition. Blackwell Science London: 406 – 407

Lewis JA, Cohen SM (2004). Addressing lead toxicity, complexation of lead ii with thopyrone and hydroxypyridine – O, S – mixed chelators. *Inorganic Chemistry* 43: 6534 – 6546.

Liu X, Song Q, Yang Y, Li W, Xu J, Wu J, Wang F, Brookes PC (2013). Human health risk assessment of heavy metals in soil-vegetable system: A multi-medium analysis. *Science of Total Environment*; 463: 530 – 640.

Ma J, Kannam K, Cheng J, Horii Y, Wu Q, Wang W (2008). Concentrations, profile and estimated human exposures for polychlorinated dibenzo-P-dioxins and dibenzo-furans from electronic waste recycling facilities and a chemical industry complex in Eastern China. *Environ Sci. Technol.* 42: 8252 – 8259.

Maduabuchi J.MU, Nzegwu CN, Adigba EO, Aloke RU, Ezomike CN, Okocha CE, Obi E, Orisakwe OE (2006). lead and cadmium exposures from canned and non-canned beverages in Nigeria: A Public Health Concern. *Science of the Total Environment.* 366: 621 – 626.

Manto WI, Angle CR, Stanek KL, Kuntzelman D, Reese YR, Kuehnemann TJ (2003). Release of lead from bone in pregnancy and lactation. *Environ Res.* 92 (2): 139 – 151.

Mendola P, Messer LC, Rappazzo K (2008). Science linking environmental contaminant exposure with fertility and reproductive health impacts in the adult female. *Fertility and Sterility.* 89 (2): e81 – e94.

Min K-B, Mina J-Y, Chos I, Kim H, Pack DY (2008). Relationship between low blood levels and growth in children of white-collar civil servants in Korea. *Int. J. Hyg. Environ. Health*; 211: 82 -87.

National Research Council (NRC 1993). Measuring lead exposure in infants, children and other sensitive population. Washington, DC: National Academy Press.

Nduka JK, Nwaro CJ, Ezenwa TE (2008b). Occupational exposure to lead poisoning, a public health concern. 31st International and Annual Conference of the Chemical Society of Nigeria. 22nd – 26th Sept. 2008. *Book of Proceedings*, 695 – 697.

Nduka JK, Odibe IO, Orisakwe OE, Ukaegbu LD, Sokcibe C (2015). Human health risk assessment of heavy metals in cosmetics in Nigeria. J.Soc. Cosmetic Chemist (In Press).

Nduka JK, Orisakwe OE (2009). Effect of effluent from Warri refinery and petrochemical company (WRPC) on water and soil qualities of contiguous host and impacted on communities of Delta state, Nigeria. *The Open Environmental Pollution and Toxicology Journal.* 1: 11 – 17.

Nduka JK, Orisakwe OE (2010). Assessment of environmental distribution of lead in some municipalities of South Eastern Nigeria. *Int. J. Environ. Res.* Public Health; 7: 2501 -2513.

Nduka JK, Orisakwe OE, Okerulu OE (2010). Heavy metal levels in muscles of some fish species from Aladja river, Warri. Nigeria: A public health concern. *Advances in Environmental Biology*; 4 (5): 125 – 130.

Nduka JKC, Orisakwe OE, Ezenweke LO, Chendo MN, Ezenwa TE (2008). Heavy metal contamination of foods by refuse dump sites in Awka, Southeastern Nigeria. *The Scientific World Journal*. 8: 941 – 948.

Nduka JKC, Constance C, Obiakor E (2006). Selective bio-accumulation of metals by different parts of some fish species from crude oil polluted water bull. Environ. Contan. Toxico. 77 (6): 846 – 853.

Nduka JKC, Orisakwe OE (2007). Heavy metal levels and physico-chemical quality of potable water supply in Warri, Nigeria. Annali di Chemica. 97 (9): 867 – 874.

Nduka JKC, Orisakwe OE, Maduagwuna CA (2008). Lead levels in paint flakes from buildings in Nigeria: A preliminary study. *Toxicology and Industrial Health*; 24: 539 – 542.

Neal AP, Guilarte TR (2012). Mechanisms of heavy metal neurotoxicity: Lead and manganese. *J. Drug Metabol and Toxicol.* S5: 002. doi: 10.4172/2157-7609.S5-002

Needdleman HL, Belinger D (1991). The health effects of low level exposure to lead. *Annu. Rev. Public Health;* 12: 111 – 140.

Needleman HL (1993). The current status of childhood low-level lead toxicity. *Neurotoxicol;* 14: 161 – 166.

Nriagu JO (1978). The biogeochemistry of lead in the environment Elsevier/North Holland. Biomedical Press: Amsterdam. The Netherlands; Part A, 138 – 164.

Nriagu JO (1979). Global inventory of natural and anthropogenic emissions of trace metals to the atmosphere. *Nature* (London); 279: 408 – 411.

Nriagu JO (1989). A global assessment of natural and source of atmospheric trace metals. *Nature* (London); 338: 48 – 49.

Nriagu JO, Afeicha M, Arowolo T, Ana G, Sridhar M, Obi E, Ebenebe J, Orisakwe O (2008). Lead poisoning associated with malaria in children of urban areas of Nigeria. *Int. J. Hyg. Environ. Health*. 211: 591 - 605.

Nriagu JO, Blankson MI, Ocran K (1996). Childhood lead poisoning in Africa: A growing public health problem. *Sci. Total Environ*; 181: 93 – 100.

Obi E, Akunyili D, Ekpo E, Orisakwe O (2006). Heavy metal hazards of Nigerian herbal remedies. *Sci. Total Environ*. 369: 35 – 41.

Onianwa PC, Adetola IG, Igwegbue CMA, Ojo MF, Tella OO (1999). Trace heavy metal composition of some Nigerian beverages and food drinks. *Food Chemistry*; 66: 275 – 279.

Orisakwe OE (2009). Environmental pollution and blood lead levels in Nigeria: Who is exposed? *Int. Journal Occup . Env. Health*. 15 (3): 315 – 317.

Orisakwe OE, Akah PA, Orish CN (1994). Prevalence of parental administration of drugs to children before coming to the hospital. *Trop. Doc.* 24: 182 – 183.

Orisakwe OE, Asomugha R, Obi E, Nduka JC, Dioka CE (2004). Impact of effluents from cable manufacturing plant on food, water and soil qualities in Nnewi, Nigeria. Pakistan. *J. Biol. Sci.* 8: 744 – 747.

Orisakwe OE, Dioke CE, Nwobodo EO, Okonkwo VC, Anike IC, Enendu AO (1996). Respiratory Abnormalities associated with occupational exposure to particulate insults in "okada" (motorcycle) operators in Nnewi. *Nig. Med. Pract.* 32: 36 – 38.

Orisakwe OE, Frazzolic C (2010). Electronic revolution and electronic wasteland: The west/waste African experience. *J. Nat. Env. Sci.* 1 (1): 43 – 47.

Orisakwe OE, Igwilo IO, Afonne OJ, Maduabuchi J-MU, Obi E, Nduka JC (2006). Heavy metal hazards of sachet water in Nigeria. Arch. Environ. Occup. Health. 61 (5): 209 – 213.

Orisakwe OE, Nduka JK (2009). Lead and cadmium levels of commonly administered pediatric syrups in Nigeria: A public health concern. *Science of the Total Environment*; 407: 5993 – 5996.

Osmond DL, Line DE, Gale JA, Gannon RW, Knott CB, Barthenhagen KA, Turnern MH, Coffey SW, Spooner J, Wells j, Walker JC, Hangroovc LL, Foster MA, Robillard PD, Lehning DW (1995). WATERSHEDSS. Water, soil and hydro-environmental decision support system. http://h20sparc.wq.ncsu.ed (Assessed January 3rd, 2009).

Pfitzner MA, Thacher TD, Petifor JM, Zoakah Al, Lawason JO, Fischer PR (2000). Prevalence of elevated blood lead levels in Nigerian children. *Ambut Child Health;* 6: 115 – 123.

Pounds JG, Long GJ, Rosen JF (1991). Cellular and molecular toxicity of lead in bone. *Environ Health Perspect.* 91: 17 – 32.

Pounds JG, Marlar RJ, Allen JR (1978). Metabolism of lead – 210 in juvenile and adults rhesus monkeys (Macaca Mulatta). *Bull Environ Contam Toxicol.* 19: 684 -691.

Pruss-Ustun A, Corvalan C (2006). Preventing disease through healthy environment: Towards an estimate of the environmental burden of disease. World Health Organisation: Geneva.

Pruvot C, Douay F, Herve F, Waterlot C (2006). Heavy metals in soil, crops and grass as a source of human exposure in the former mining areas. *Journal of Soils and Sediments.* 6 (4): 215 – 220.

Qian ZM, Xiao DS, Wang Q, Tang PL, Pu YM (1997). Inhibitory mechanism of lead on transferrin-bond iron uptake by rabbit reticulocytes: A fractal analysis. *Mol. Cell. Biochem.* 173: 89 – 94.

Rabinowitz M, Wetherill GW, Kopple JD (1974). Studies of human lead metabolism by use of stable isotope tracers. *Environ Health Perspect.* 7: 145 -152.

Rogan W, Ware J (2007). Exposure to lead in children – how low is low enough? *New Engl. J. Med.* 348 (16): 1515 – 1516.

Schmidt CW (2006). Unfair trade, e-waste in Africa. Environ. Health Perspect; 144: A232 – A235.

Soldina OP, Miller M, Soldin SJ (2003). Pediatric reference ranges for zinc protoporphyrin. *Clin. Biochem.* 36: 21 – 25.

Stone R (2009). Science 325.1055. U.S. environmental protection agency. characterization of products containing lead and cadmium in municipal solid waste in the United States. 1970 to 2000; EPA/530-SW-89-015B; Office of Solid Waste: Washington, DC, 1989.

Sun C-C, Wong T-T, Hwang Y-H, Chao K-Y, Jee S-H, Wang J-D (2002). "Percutaneous absorption of inorganic lead compounds". American Industrial Hygiene Association Journal. 63 (5): 641 – 646.

U.S. Department of Energy (2004). RAIS. Risk assessment information system. http://risk.isd.ornl/gov/rap_hpshtml

U.S. Environmental Protection Agency (1989). Risk assessment guidance for superfund. Vol 1: Human Health Evaluation Manual EPA/540/1-89/002. Office of Solid Waste and Emergency Response. U.S. Environmental Protection Agency. Washington D.C. http://www.epa/gov/superfund programs risk/ragsa/index.htm

U.S. Environmental Protection Agency (1996). soil screening guidance. technical background document. EPA/540/R-95128. Office of Solid Waste and Emergency Response. U.S. Environmental Protection Agency. Washington D.C. http://www.epa.gov/superfund resource/soil/toc.htmllpl

U.S. Environmental Protection Agency (2001). Supplemental guidance for developing soil screening levels for superfund sites. OSWER 93554-24. Office of Solid Waste and Emergency Response. U.S. Environmental Protection agency Washington. D.C. http://www.epa.gov/superfund/ resources/soil/ssgmarchol.pdf.

US Environmental Protection Agency (EPA 1989). Evaluation of the potential carcinogenicity of lead and lead compounds. office of health and environmental assessment; EPA/600/8-89/045A.

US EPA (2011). Section 2.4.1.1, Pages 51589 – 51590 of the HRS rule. http://ww.epa.gov/superfund/training/hrstrain/htmain/s2411.htm. (Assessed Oct. 08 2014).

Van den Berg R (1995). Human exposure to soil contamination: A qualitative and quantitative analysis towards proposals for human toxicology intervention values. RIVM Report no. 725201011 National Institute of Public Health and Environmental Protection (RIVM) Bilthoven. The Netherlands. http://www.nvm.nl.bibliotheck rapporten.725201011.html

Vupputuri S, He J, Muntner P, Bazzano LA, Whelton PK, Batuman V (2003). Blood lead level is associated with elevated blood pressure in blacks. Hypertens; 41: 463 – 468.

Wallace B, Cooper K (1986). The citizens guide to lead: Uncovering a hidden health hazard; NC Press Ltd: Toronto, Canada.

Wells AC, Venn JB, Heard MJ (1975). Deposition in the lung and uptake to blood of motor exhaust labelled with 203Pb. Inhaled Part 4 Pt. 1: 175 – 189.

White C, Masanet E, Rosen C, Beckman SJ (2003). *Cleaner Prod.* 11: 445 – 458.

WHO Media Centre (2008). Traditional medicine. Factsheet N^{A} 134. 2008. (http://ww.who.int/mediacentre/factsheet/fs134/en/), (Accessed June 2011).

Wright N, Thatcher TD, pfitzner MA, Fischer PR, Petitor JM (2005). Causes of lead toxicity in a Nigerian city. *Arch. Dis. Child*; 90: 262 – 266.

Yule W, Rutter M (1985). Effect on children's behaviour and cognitive performance: A critical review. In Mahaffrey R. (ed). Dietary and Environment Lead: Human Health Services, New York. NY: Elsevier; 211 – 251.

Zhou F, Guo HC, Liu L (2007). Quantitative identification and source apportionment of anthropogenic heavy metals in marine of Hong Kong. *Environmental Geology*. 53: 295 – 305.

Ziegler EE, Edwards BB, Jensen RL, Maharffey KR, Fomon SJ (1978). Absorption and retention of lead by infants. *Pediatr. Res*. 12: 29 – 34.

In: Lead Exposure and Poisoning
Editor: Leonard Horton
ISBN: 978-1-63482-699-0

Chapter III

Changes in Intestinal Microflora in Rats Induced by Oral Exposure to Low Lead (II) Concentrations

Ilya Digel**, Rustam Sadykov, Aysegül Artmann and Gerhard Artmann

Institute of Bioengineering, Aachen University of Applied Sciences, Juelich, Germany

Abstract

Soluble forms of lead Pb(II) are well known toxins, entering organisms of humans and animals predominantly orally. Intestinal microflora represents a necessary functional component of the body and, together with intestinal epithelium, is usually subjected to the highest Pb(II) concentrations. This implies the importance of detailed study of lead impact in this particular context.

* Corresponding author: Dr. Ilya Digel. Laboratory of Cell- and Microbiology, Institute for Bioengineering, Aachen University of Applied Sciences, FB9, Heinrich-Mussmann-Str. 1, 52428 Jülich, Germany. Tel.: +49 (0)241600953862, e-mail: digel@fh-aachen.de.

The aim of our study was to investigate the influence of lead at different doses on the structure of the intestinal microbial community *in vivo* (rat) and its relationships to intestinal epithelium *in vitro*. In our experiments, lead doses that were much lower than those causing visible harmful effects on cell culture or on the level of the whole body, induced significant changes in intestinal microflora. Oral exposure to Pb created selective advantages for lactose-negative coli-forms and thus contributed into dysbacteriosis development. We suppose that the lead-induced dysbacteriosis was initiated by the changes in bacterial adhesion to the intestinal epithelium. This might be related to increased intestinal epithelium permeability also caused by lead, as it was shown in another series of our studies shown here. Furthermore, model dynamic light scattering measurements have revealed strong aggregating effect of lead on protein (albumin) solutions.

The results could be possibly extrapolated to human beings, opening the opportunity to understand some mysterious cases of persisting dysbacteriosis as a result of latent Pb-intoxication. This, in turn, suggests a probiotic treatment as a promising therapy for lead-exposed patients on one hand and possible success of Pb-scavenging therapy for some patients with dysbacteriosis on the other hand.

Keywords: dysbacteriosis, IEC-6, intestinal microflora, lead toxicity, rat

Introduction

Soluble lead Pb (II) is one of the oldest known and most studied occupational and environmental toxins. Decades of use of lead-based paints and leaded gasoline have resulted in widespread contamination. Although lead has been later eliminated from household use, its compounds are still widely used in industrial processes and products [1, 2].

Pb mainly affects the nervous system [3], blood and blood-forming organs, kidneys and gastrointestinal tract [4, 5]. The problem of lead presence in drinking water [6] and in airborne particles [7] remains acute in many countries. There is no apparent threshold for lead toxicity [8], suggesting that several different pathological mechanisms are involved.

Despite intensive study, there is still vigorous debate about the toxic effects of lead, mainly concerning low-level exposure in the general population owing to environmental pollution by lead alone and in combination with other compounds [9, 10].

Total Pb dietary intake for an adult may vary from 20 to 150 μg per day in most countries with maximal daily dose of 0.2-2 mg regarded as safe [11, 12]. The main routes of lead entrance into the human body (food, water, dust) involve the intestinal system. Young children are especially susceptible to lead poisoning because they have 4–5 times higher intestinal absorption [1].

Lead absorption is significantly influenced by the dietary intakes of iron, calcium, phosphorus, pectin etc., and has been reviewed extensively [13-17]. The most easily accessible forms of lead are acetate, chloride and tetraethyl, whereas in the intestine, lead is mainly bound to bile acids (cholic and chenodeoxycholic) that contribute to lead transportation (translocation) in the intestinal epithelium [18]. Unabsorbed lead is excreted with feces.

Some direct pathological effects of high doses of lead on the intestinal system have been mentioned in the literature and were attributed to dilation of the gastric mucosal microcirculation accompanied by desquamation of surface mucous cells [19]. It also has been reported also that lead acts as a chemical stressor and causes the breakdown of the homeostatic cellular mechanisms [20].

The fact that intestinal microflora is usually subjected to the highest Pb concentrations in the body implies the importance of more detailed study of lead impact in this particular context. The human gastrointestinal tract displays an enormous variety of both aerobic and anaerobic microbial species. Some 900-1000 species belonging mainly to the *Escherichia, Bacteroides, Bifidobacterium, Lactobacillus* genera that encode about 5 million genes have been identified so far [21]. In spite of many individual contributing factors (diet, physical activity, etc.), the microbiome is practically stable in healthy adults and plays a role in the maintenance of a healthy state.

While the contribution of the indigenous gut microbial community to the healthy state is widely recognized, only recently has there been evidence pointing to indigenous flora in disease. Apparently, alterations in the composition of the gut microbiome lead to pathological dysbiosis, and have been related to an increasing number of intestinal and extra-intestinal diseases [21]. In 2004 F. Savino with and colleagues has reported that changes in gut microflora could play an important role in the pathogenesis of infantile colic, a common problem in the first months of life [22]. Since then, evidence is growing that environmentally caused perturbations of intestinal host-microbe interactions can lead to miscues and altered host responses that increase the risk of pathogenic processes and promote "western" disorders such as inflammatory bowel diseases, cancers, obesity, diabetes, autism, and asthma [23]. Changes in microbe-host relationships and following resulting abnormal expansion of gut microbial flora into the small bowel or small intestinal bacterial overgrowth are now known causes of acute pancreatitis, bacterial gastroenteritis, irritable bowel syndrome, and many other diseases [24].

In spite of its obvious importance, the influence of sub-chronic intestinal lead exposure on the intestinal microbial community and its relationships with intestinal epithelium are still underestimated and poorly studied.

This is also true for many dietary toxins, for which the study of the pathological effects is focused predominantly on host tissues and cells, but totally neglects the responses from commensal microbial flora.

The aim of the present study was to investigate the influence of lead at different doses on the structure of the rat intestinal microbial community *in vivo* and its relationships to intestinal epithelium *in vitro*. We also have attempted to address possible molecular mechanisms of the observed phenomena. The understanding of the underlying role of altered commensal gut microbiota in dietary toxicity could lead to novel diagnostic and therapeutic strategies and would appreciably contribute to public health.

Materials and Methods

Reagents

As a source of lead, soluble Pb salts (lead (II) acetate and lead (II) chloride) were used. There were two main reasons for not using more "natural" cholic acid-group Pb compounds in our study. First, these substances show significant self-aggregation and sturdy binding to the plastic and glassware surfaces that would make the correct dosage virtually impossible the correct dosage at very low Pb concentrations. Second, better comparability and interpretation of the obtained data were pursued, since most existing literature sources on the topic deal with the chloride and acetate force source of lead. The Pb(II) concentrations used in the experiments were calculated based on available lead toxicity data obtained from reference books and material safety data sheets (MSDS) provided by manufacturers [1, 2, 8, 25, 26]. In the case of oral administration, the 50% lethal dose LD_{50} (rat) was assumed to be 4.665 mg/kg for lead acetate $Pb(CH_3COO)_2$ (trihydrate form). In some experiments, sodium chloride and sodium acetate were used as a control, in addition to the main "blanc" controls (isotonic buffered saline). All chemicals used were reagent grade and purchased from Sigma-Aldrich Chemie GmbH, Taufkirchen, Germany.

Animal Experiments

White outbred adult male rats with a body mass of 180-220 g used for the experiments were obtained from the Biology Faculty's vivarium of Al-Farabi Kazakh National University (Almaty).

The experimental groups and the concentrations of lead were chosen to give maximum information from a reasonable number of experiments. The rats were separated into one control and 4 experimental groups, with 3 rats in each group. All the animals were maintained on a standard laboratory diet ("Regal Rat" rat fodder), under the same standard conditions. The "ad libitum" feeding regimen was used. The first experimental group received 1/14 of oral LD_{50} (corresponding to 333.21 mg/kg body weight) every day for 2 weeks. The second, third and fourth experimental groups received 1/60 (77.75 mg/kg), 1/240 (19.44 mg/kg), and 1/960 (4.86 mg/kg), of LD_{50}, respectively. The lead acetate water solution (1 ml) was administered orally, once a day, using a plastic syringe with a catheter. The control group was administered 1 ml of sterile isotonic NaCl solution.

Before the actual experiments began, the fecal samples of all rats were collected for preliminary microbiological and chemical analyses. Further samples were taken every day during the whole period of lead administration (14 days). After 2 weeks of lead exposure, the animals were euthanized by carbon dioxide inhalation [27]. The whole gastrointestinal tract from the lower esophagus to the colon was removed. Blood and organs (large and small intestine, stomach, kidneys and liver) were separately analyzed for lead content using atomic absorption spectrometry.

All animal procedures in this study were carried out by licensed investigators and in accordance with regulated procedures under the Animals (Scientific Procedures) Act (1986).

Microbiological Analysis

A common criterion for bacterial viability is the ability to reproduce in a suitable nutrient medium (colony forming unit (CFU) counting,). For analysis of microbial flora present in excreta, samples of known mass containing different concentrations of Pb were collected individually from each rat (3 fecal samples from a single rat, 3 rats in a group) and transferred under sterile conditions into clean glass tubes. After that, the feces were thoroughly homogenized in sterile phosphate-buffered saline (PBS; pH 7.4, 1:9, w/v) and serial 10× dilutions were made to obtain 10^3, 10^5 and 10^7 times diluted working solutions. From every dilution, 100 μL were transferred into a Petri dish containing selective agar culture medium and spread out by a glass spatula. The media used were: Endo agar (for isolation and identification of *E. coli*), MRS agar (for *Lactobacillus sp.*) and Sabouraud agar (for yeasts).

The media were purchased from Lab M company (International Diagnostics Group, Lancashire, United Kingdom). The Petri dishes containing MRS agar were placed into specialized exsiccators to create anaerobic conditions. After incubation at 37°C for 24-48 hours, bacterial colonies were counted (using a "blind" method to avoid subjective bias in the results caused by experimenter's intent) and additionally identified using light microscopy and corresponding microbiological staining. If the number of colonies ranged between 10 and 800 per Petri plate, the data were included in the results. The successful counts of the colonies were further calculated as concentrations of colony-forming units per gram of fecal mass.

Atomic Absorption Spectrometry

The concentration of lead in organs and excreta was determined by means of using the atomic absorption spectrometer AAS-1N (Carl Zeiss Co, Jena, Germany) according to the standard measurement protocol [28]. In brief, 500 mg of homogenized sample was mixed in a quartz glass with 25 ml of concentrated nitric acid and 25 ml of double-distilled water, boiled, cooled down and mixed with 5% nitric acid to a final volume of 10 ml. The sample was placed in the atomic absorption spectrometer and ignited in a propane-air flame. The lead-specific 283.3 nm absorption was measured and compared to known standard values.

Adhesion Assay

The bacterial strains used in the adhesion experiments were *Lactobacillus plantarum* subsp. *plantarum* (ATCC 14917, serological group D), and *Escherichia coli* (ATCC 15223 serotype O13:H11, Lac^- (i^+ z^+ y^-)-mutable).

The microorganisms were cultured in liquid culture media (MRS and Trypton Soy Broth, respectively) to reach the appropriate amount of biomass, washed 2 two times with sterile phosphate-buffered saline (PBS; pH 7.4) and kept suspended in PBS until the experiments began.

As a model of intestinal epithelium, the normal rat epithelial cells IEC-6 from the small intestine were used. Many aspects of the distribution and concentration of lead in animals resemble the distribution of lead in the human body [19].

Intestine and intestinal epithelial cells of rats have become of great interest and show the validity of using them as a model to study the toxic effect of lead on the intestine.

However, it should be kept in mind that, for example, the lead absorption coefficient is slightly different (0.36±0.07 for humans and 0.23±0.020 in rats) [29-31].

The IEC-6 cells were obtained from the German Collection of Microorganisms and Cell Cultures (DSMZ). They are adherent, transparent, epitheloid cells growing as monolayers (displaying polymorphy of cell forms). They represent a non-continuous cell line with usually about 10-15 doublings and are able to synthesize fibronectin and collagen [32]. After thawing of the stock (stored in liquid nitrogen), the IEC-6 were cultured in 45% Dulbecco's medium (DMEM) containing 4.5 g/L glucose with addition of 45% RPMI 1640, 10% fetal bovine serum and 0.1 U/mL insulin. To obtain the necessary amount of biomass, the confluent cultures were split from 1:2 to 1:4 about twice a week using trypsin/EDTA, seeded out at approx. 3-6 x 10^5 cells/25 cm^2 and incubated at 37°C with 5% CO_2.

For adhesion studies, the confluent monolayer of cells (5th passage) was grown in 35 mm×10 mm plastic chambers with Nunclon Surface (Nunc GmbH, Wiesbaden, Germany) in 2 ml of DMEM. Four-day post-confluent IEC-6 monolayers were washed twice with 1 mL of sterile DMEM (without Phenol Red indicator) before the adhesion assay.

The amount of attached bacteria depended on their initial concentration; therefore, the same final dilution of bacterial suspension was used for all experimental groups, allowing only the Pb concentration to vary between the groups. Since the lactic acid bacteria have a tendency to form chains and aggregates that make visual counting difficult, in this study the microplate method was adopted instead. After 24 h incubation of the monolayer with culture medium containing different concentrations of lead acetate, the cells were washed twice with 2 ml of pure DMEM.

After that, 1ml of the test bacteria suspensions at concentrations between 10^5 and 10^8 CFU/ ml were added to 1 ml of complete culture medium. This suspension (2 ml) was added to each chamber and incubated for 1 hour at 37°C, in a 5% CO_2 atmosphere, with gentle rocking. After that, the medium with non-adhered bacterial cells was collected from each chamber into 3 microplate wells (200 μL each) and the cell concentration was measured at 490 nm using a microplate reader (Bio-Rad Co. US). A lower optical density was interpreted as a lower concentration of bacterial cell, and thus, as a caseindicative of better adhesion [33].

For each concentration of lead (II) acetate, 3 plastic chambers were used. Control groups (each in triplicate) were created for adhesion experiments. In the first group, pure medium without microbial cells was added to the IEC-6 monolayer to check the contribution of the adhered cells alone to the photometric signal. In the second group, the microbial suspension was added into a plastic chamber without cells to take into account the nonunspecific adhesion of bacteria to plastic surface. Finally, the optical density of the native microbial suspension was measured to establish the initial reference point.

At the end of the adhesion experiments, after the samples had been taken for optical density measurements, the monolayers were washed twice with sterile PBS (pH 7.4), fixed with methanol, Giemsa stained, and examined microscopically [33]. Additional visual counting of adhered cells was conducted in triplicate by two people and the number of adherent bacteria was counted ondetermined to be about 1,000 IEC-6 cells, in 50 randomly selected microscopic fields.

Permeability Measurement Setup and Procedure

IEC-6 permeability was measured with the setup shown in Figure 1 at in vitro conditions after incubation with different doses of lead (II) acetate as compared to the control groups (without treatment).

The measurement system was specially designed to address the permeability of thin films or confluent cell monolayers and allowed the real-time detection of the permeability [34]. Since diffusion measurements are temperature-dependent, the whole system was permanently keptconsitently maintained at 37±1°C.

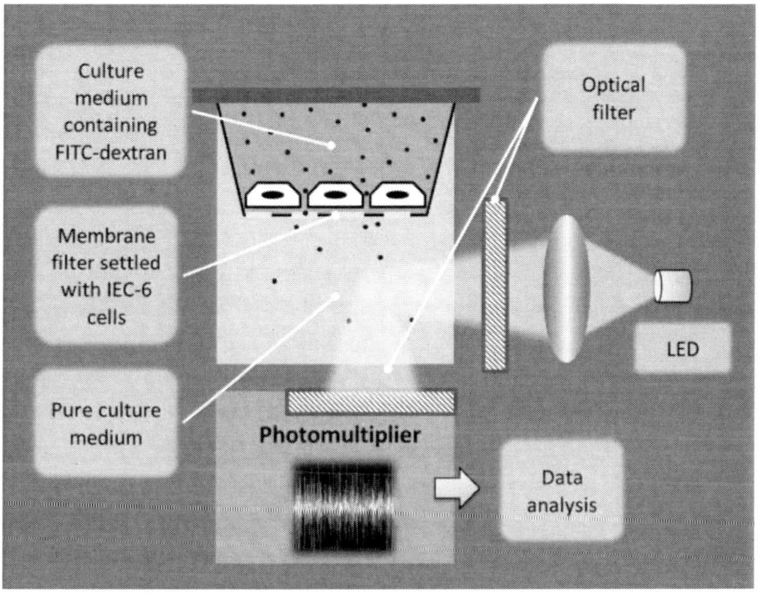

Figure 1. Setup for IEC-6 monolayer permeability measurement.

In brief, the device consists of a specially designed rotary table with holes for quartz cuvettes (12 pieces), in which filters settled with cells can be installed. Intestinal epithelial cells were first cultured on the top of Falcon filters (Beston Dickenson and Co. US, pore size 1 μm), in 2 mL of culture medium (DMEM), until a confluent cell monolayer was achieved. Next, cells were exposed to various doses (0.1 nM – 10 μM) of lead acetate for 24 hours. In control samples, equivalent amount of sodium acetate was added.

The experiments were conducted with fluorescein isothiocyanate labeled dextran (FITC-dextan, 10.5 kDa) as the diffusing and measured compound. The Ffluorescence signal was measured with a photomultiplier at 519 nm, upon using 495 nm wavelength for excitation. The intensity of the emitted light was directly proportional to the amount of FITC-dextran having passed through the membrane. Due to the FITC-dextran diffusion through the cellular monolayer, the fluorescence intensity increases with time in an exponential manner: $I = e^{Pt}$, where P value can be considered as a "permeability coefficient," characterizing the rate of diffusion [34].

Dynamic Light Scattering Measurements of Bovine Serum Albumin Aggregation

Dynamic light scattering (DLS) data were obtained with a temperature-controlled DAWN-EOS instrument equipped with quasi-elastic LS module (Wyatt Technology Corp., Santa Barbara, US) at 37°C. Temperature variations during a single measurement never exceeded ± 0.2°C.

The instrument was used in batch (not flow-through) mode using glass scintillation cells filled bubble-free with a 4mL protein sample. Bovine serum albumin, (BSA) "Fraction V" was purchased from Sigma-Aldrich Co. (Munich, Germany). The working BSA solution (1 mg/mL) was prepared using a phosphate buffered saline, PBS (P5368 Sigma-Aldrich Co.), in a dust-free environment. For the measurement, 6 mL of the working solution were filtered through 0.2 μm Whatman nitrocellulose membrane filter into a QELS glass scintillation vial (Wheaton, US) using a one-way plastic syringe. The pH value 7.4±0.2, osmolarity and the BSA concentration in the samples have been kept constant throughout all measurements.

The time-dependent autocorrelation function (ACF) of the photon current was monitored with a software correlator provided by the manufacturer. The first sampling time was 0.96 μs. ACFs were taken and sampled every 2 s, containing 105 to 106 counts each. Sets of collected ACFs were averaged and stored for analysis. Light scattering data analysis was performed by means of Astra® software (Wyatt Technology Corp., Santa Barbara, US) using a second-order cumulant function [35]. In this case, the basic formula relates the hydrodynamic radius Rh to the first cumulant, Γ1 is:

$$Rh = kBTq2 / 6\pi\eta\Gamma1 \text{ where } q2 = (4\pi ns / \lambda0) \sin(\Theta/2)$$

where **q** is the scattering vector, $\boldsymbol{\lambda_0}$ is the vacuum wavelength of incident light, $\boldsymbol{n_s}$ is the index of refraction of the solution, **Θ** is the scattering angle, $\boldsymbol{k_B}$ is the Boltzmann constant, and **η** is the solvent viscosity at the experimental Kelvin temperature ***T***. The sample polydispersity was computed from $P=\Gamma_2/(\Gamma_1)^2$. This quantity was used for discarding data that showed values of $p > 0.05$, indicating excessive noise due to aggregates or dust. The radius was corrected for the refractive index, assuming $n = 1.329$ for water at 783 nm [36].

During the protein aggregation measurement runs, freshly prepared Pb(II) acetate stock solution was injected through a 0.2 μm Whatman filter into the scintillation vial containing the sample to achieve the desired working concentration (1 μM or 1 mM). In the control group measurement, the same working molar concentration of sodium acetate was achieved.

Results and Discussion

As shown in Figure 2, in our experiments the amount of accumulated lead in rat organs changed roughly proportionally to the received dose, mainly concentrated in the kidneys and large intestine. Small amounts of lead were detected even in the presumably "clean" control group, indicating background lead consumption via drinking water, air dust and fodder.

The lowest administered dose of the lead used in these experiments 1/960 LD_{50} (corresponds to 4.86 mg/kg) caused minor shifts in concentrations of lead in the organs but did not visibly influence its distribution.

Further increases in the administered amount of lead resulted in more significant rise of its detectable concentration first in kidneys and then in the digestive organs.

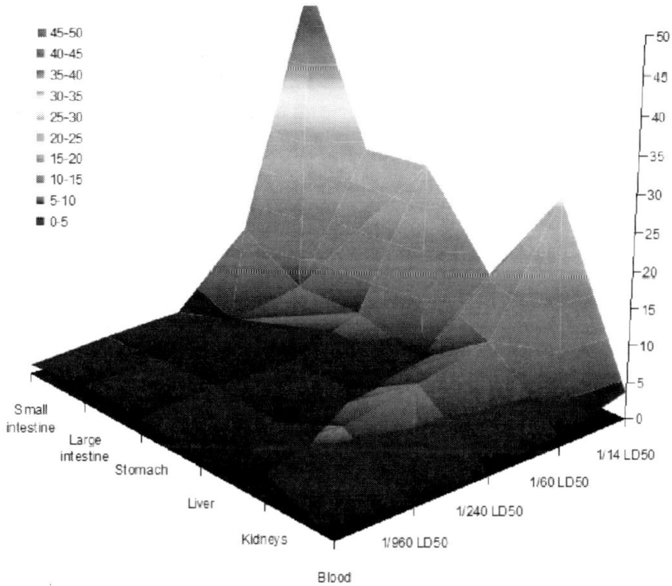

The concentrations are given as fractions of LD50, which corresponds to 4.66 mg/g of body mass.

Figure 2. Lead distribution in rat organs after 1 week of oral lead intake measured by atomic absorption spectrometry.

The collation of the data in Figure 2 with the daily Pb amount measured in rat feces during a 2-week period of time (data not shown here) implied the constant increase of inter-intestinal Pb concentration even in the case of the lowest dose given. Higher Pb concentrations caused proportionally higher rates of the of Pb accumulation. The data shown in Figure 2, obtained using atomic absorption spectrometry, are in agreement with those previously reported by K. Kostial, I. Simonovic, and M. Pisonic, who used ^{203}Pb labelling for lead intestinal absorption measurements [37].

However, specific mechanisms of lead action on intestinal epithelial cells are still poorly understood. Considering the intestinal absorption as a limiting factor for lead transport to other organs it was interesting to examine the effects of lead on intestinal permeability level.

As an in-vitro intestinal epithelium model, we used a confluent layer of intestinal epithelial cells IEC-6, as described in the methods section. Figure 3 presents data on the permeability of the IEC-6 monolayer under influence of various doses of lead (II) acetate to intestinal epithelial cells.

The lead exposure in small doses apparently affected intercellular junctions, resulting in appreciable permeability increase corresponding to the received dose of lead. An even more dramatic increase in the permeability of cell monolayers of IEC-6 observed upon usage of even higher doses of lead (1μM - 10 μM), can presumably be presumably associated with the emergence of a cytotoxic effect that was visible ion microscopic photos.

Quite similar effects on (capillary) permeability have been reported by Struzynska with coworkers - in their study inorganic Pb(II) administered at low doses, induced blood-brain barrier dysfunction [38].

More detailed information on about particular molecular interactions involved into permeability changes induced by heavy metals is becoming available. In 2013 S. Boucherie et al., have showed that changes induced by cadmium on the cell-cell junctions in hepatocytes are related to Cx32/claudin 2.

The exact mechanisms of the epithelial permeability changes induced by lead are yet to be studied. Therefore, upcoming actualization of concepts in the intestinal toxicology of Pb must include advances in understanding the mechanisms and cellular specificity of Pb.

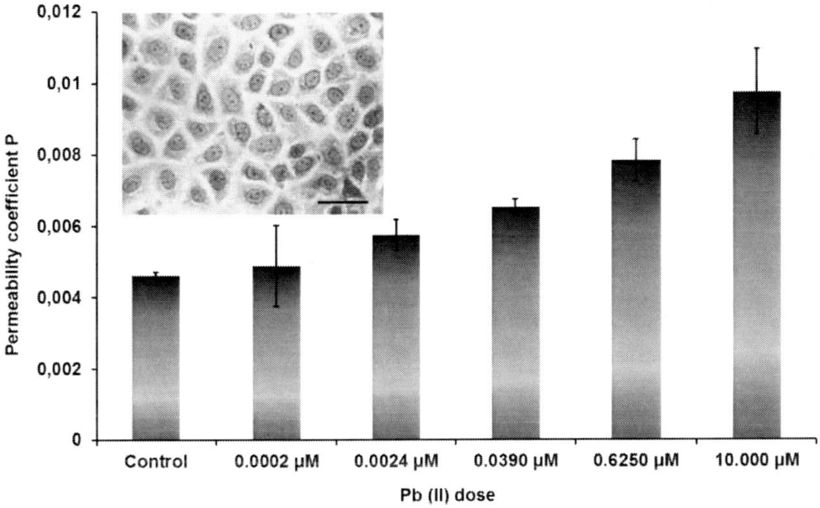

The photo shows a fragment of confluent layer of ICES-6 cells formed on the membrane after vital staining with Giemsa dye (scale bar 100 μm). Sample number n=6 for each dose.

Figure 3. Effect of different doses of lead (II) acetate on IEC-6 permeability measured after 24 h of incubation.

In our opinion, two potential routes of toxic action need to be considered primarily: (1) direct Pb(II) binding with the tight-junction complexes and (2) its indirect action from inside the cell, by alternation of cytoskeletal pathways.

Conscerning the processes induced by lead in intestinal microflora, the changes observed in the relative amount of lactose-positive lac(+) and lactose-negative lac(-) *E. coli* cells as a reaction to elevated Pb concentration (Figure 4) were most drastic dramatic and interesting.

The fermentation of lactose is a diagnostic characteristic of *Escherichia coli*; however, nonfermenting mutants can readily be obtained. These mutants may show losses or changes in the accumulation of lactose or other p-galactosides in the cell, or in the formation or activity of the enzyme β-galactosidase, which splits lactose to the constituent monosaccharides. Such mutants have played an important part in the analysis of gene action by Jacob and Monod [39].

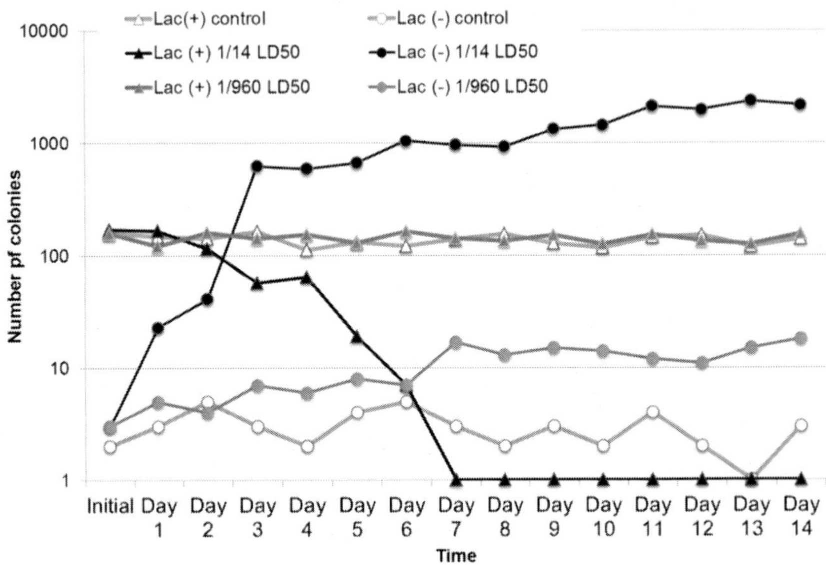

The number of colony-forming units (CFUs) was counted every day for the different concentrations of Pb administered and is shown respectively with respect to the dilution used. The number of CFU per gram corresponds to the number of colonies (y-axis) $\times 10^4$ for both lac(+) and lac(-) E. coli. The concentration of lead is given as a fractions of LD50, which corresponds to 4.665 mg/kg of rat body weight.

Figure 4. Dynamics of lac (-) (above) and lac (+) (below) E. coli in rat intestines in response to continual (2 weeks) lead (II) intake.

During the first 3-4 days of lead administration the concentration of both *E. coli* lac(-) variants did not differ between the control and the experimental groups. However, the measurements made in the following 10-12 days showed intensifying differences between lac(+) and lac(-) *E. coli* responses to Pb presence. While the lac(+) *E. coli* variants were, as expected, inhibited by the presence of Pb in a concentration-dependent manner, the lac(-) group appeared to use the weakening of competition caused by Pb to its advantage in the same concentration-dependent way. Ats the highest inter-intestinal Pb concentrations were reached (10-15 mg/g feces), the dominance of lac(-) forms was became obvious.

Figure 5 summarizes the changes induced in rat intestinal microflora after 2 weeks of continuous Pb (II) intake according to the doses given.

Though the absolute and relative amounts of different intestinal bacteria in the control group did not differ significantly after 2 weeks from the initial values (the two sets of bars on the left), even the smallest lead doses used in the experiment (4.86 mg/kg and 19.44 mg/kg, corresponding to 1/960 of LD_{50} and 1/240 of LD_{50}, respectively) resulted in distinct alterations in bacterial microflora (Figure 5, the two bar sets in the middle).

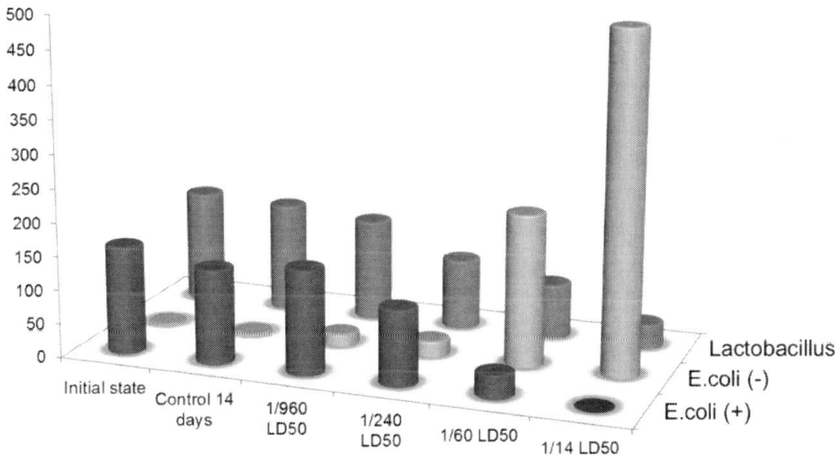

The lactose-positive (+) and negative (-) E. coli colonies are shown separately to show the impact of lead of lac-phenotype. The data is shown irrespectively to the suspension dilution used (10^4 E. coli lac(+), 10^4 E. coli lac(-), 10^7 Lactobacillus, 10^3 yeasts) in order to draw attention to the relative dynamics of the strains used.

Figure 5. Changes induced in rat intestinal microflora after 2 weeks of continuous Pb (II) intake according to the dose given. The vertical axis shows the CFU number.

For violation in of the qualitative or quantitative composition of the normal intestinal microflora F. Nissl in 1916 coined the term "*dysbiosis*" (originally regarding *E. coli* only).

According to modern concepts, intestinal dysbiosis (also termed *diysbacteriosis*) refers to general microbial imbalance on or inside the body. and isIt can be further defined as clinical and laboratory syndrome, associated with metabolic and immunological disorders with possible development of gastrointestinal disorders, such as inflammatory bowel disease, chronic fatigue syndrome, colitis, etc.

Thus, the key of a disease's origin lies on in the imbalance occurring as a result of dysregulation of (normal) bacterial antagonisms in the intestinal microbiota due to their exposure to a number of endogenous and exogenous factors.

OIn order to investigate possible reasons for the observed deep changes in the intestinal microbial community caused even by low concentrations of lead at low concentrations, we performed a series of *in vitro* experiments, using cultured rat intestinal cells, the IEC-6, and homogenous bacterial suspensions. After being brought in contact with intestinal cell monolayer, some of the applied bacteria firmly adhered to the cell surface and could be counted microscopically.

High concentrations (1.0 – 5.0 mM) of lead acetate showed show in our studies distinct cytotoxic effects on IEC-6 cells after 24 h incubation, and, therefore, were not used for adhesion studies.

The dose of lead used for adhesion experiments was in the range of 0.1 nM - 0.5 μM per chamber (2 ml), which corresponds to 50 nM - 0.25 mM concentrations in the culture medium. The adhesion of the cells was measured microscopically and spectrophotometrically.

It was found that for lactose-negative *E. coli* cells, a broad interval of lead acetate concentrations exists (2.5 - 250 μM), where the adhesion of the bacteria to intestinal cells was stimulated compared to the control [40]. The maximum of *E. coli* adsorption (approx. 105%-108% relative to the control) was observed at ~78 μM concentration (for both salts used) corresponding to the a dose of ~ 0.1565 μmol per flask.

In contrast to *E. coli*, adhesion of *Lactobacillus* cells was significantly inhibited by lead, showing some increase at only one concentration (~326 μM) which could possibly be attributable to the contribution of electrostatic interactions. Similar effects were also found when lead (II) chloride was used as a source of lead.

Probing the Interaction of Human Serum Albumin with Pb(II)

Like in the case of the observed alterations in cellular permeability, adhesion-related effects also deserve a closer look form from the molecular perspective. For instance, the understanding of lead (II) neurotoxicity has moved significantly forward due to the appreciation of intermolecular interactions that manifest themselves on the cellular level.

General consensus holds to the existence of prime target proteins for heavy metals. Lead might interfere with the physiological activity of these particularly susceptible target proteins, either by forming a complex with functional side chain groups or by displacing essential metal ions in metalloproteins [41]. Now it is becoming clear that at least some Pb-induced learning impairments and cognitive deficits are related to NMDA receptor function that, in turn, might be affected by a 78-kDa molecular chaperone glucose-regulated protein (GRP78). In vitro studies showed that Pb strongly binds to GRP78, inducing its aggregation [42].

We were wondering if the binding of Pb(II) to proteins and resulting protein aggregation reported by our colleagues [42, 43] Pb(II) -binding to proteins and following protein aggregation are protein-specific or rather more common phenomena. With this aim in view, we investigated the Pb-acetate action of bovine serum albumin (BSA) folding and aggregation by using a dynamic light scattering device. In last the past few years, we conducted numerous of studies on protein aggregation and could were able to use an elaborated setup and protocols [36, 44].

BSA was chosen as a well-studied and easily available protein of high quality for light scattering studies. First, molecular size of freshly prepared BSA in PBS buffer (1mg/mL) was measured (first 100 minutes on the Figure 6). The light scattering signal showed a typical appcarance corresponding to a ~5nm molecular radius with just a few aggregates of different size. An injection of sodium acetate (final concentration 1mM) did not result in any measurable changes in BSA molecules population (Figure 6, arrow A).

By contrast, administration of Pb acetate up to 1μM first caused surprisingly rushed sedimentation of previously suspended molecular aggregates (see clear zone following the arrow B). Further increase of Pb acetate concentration (up to 1mM) resulted in appearance of numerous molecular aggregates of BSA, with single-molecule protein fraction getting becoming almost depleted (Figure 6, right to the arrow C).

Our data suggest that serum albumins, and probably some other extra (cellular) proteins also as well, can be considered as a target for Pb binding and interactions.

To our knowledge, no such direct measurements with lead-induced protein aggregation have been ever performed. In the existing literature, scarce data on the formation of cadmium acetate HSA complexes [45] and keratin aggregation by inorganic Pb are presented [43].

However we believe that the ability of heavy metals to impede protein folding and promote protein aggregation, with followingaccompanied by dysregulation of cellular control systems resulting in misfolding disorders (including Alzheimer disease) will probably become an important topic in the coming decades [11, 41].

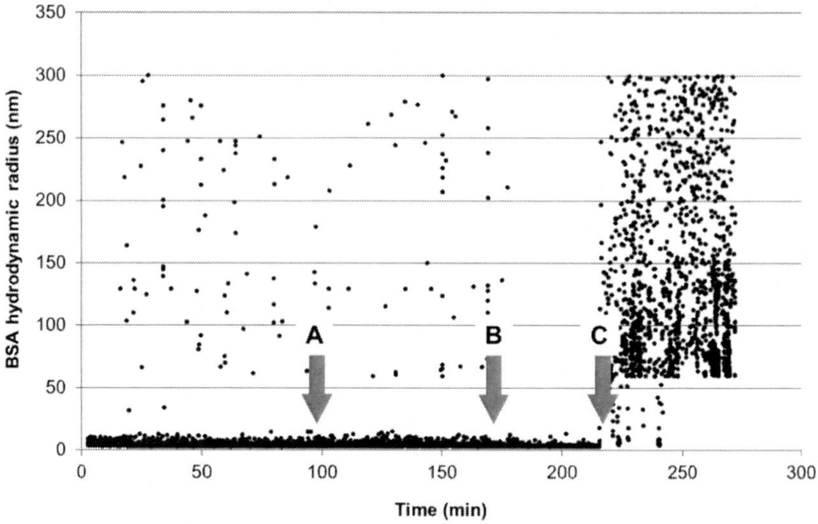

The gray arrows represent the injection events resulted in (A) 1 mM sodium acetate (B) 1 μM lead acetate and (C) 1mM lead acetate final concentrations.

Figure 6. Bovine serum albumin aggregation caused by Pb(II) detected by dynamic light scattering.

Conclusion

A great amount of research effort has been devoted to the description of intestinal absorption of heavy metals [14, 46, 47], but their effects on intestinal microflora have not drawn any serious attention. Previous studies have suggested that lead toxicity is the result of its effect on calcium metabolism [16, 17, 48], and channel dysfunction [49].

Nevertheless, the main mechanisms underlying lead toxicity at low concentrations remain unclear, maybe because of the absence of a systemic molecular approach to understanding lead toxicity.

Recent studies have revealed the intricate relationship between the vast population of microbes that live in our gut and the human host [50]. Our experiments were designed, primarily, first, to investigate the effects of lead on the rat intestinal microbial community, and secondarily, to study if whether the effect is related to microbial adhesion to rat intestinal epithelial cells.

The rat, as well as its intestinal cells, has been shown to be a good model for toxicological animal-human bioavailability correlations [29-31]. Many aspects of concentration and distribution of lead in rat resemble those in the human body. Nevertheless, some interspecies variations in intestinal absorption (0.36±0.07 for human beings and 0.23±0.02 for rats) should be taken into account.

The results of our atomic absorption spectrometry measurements of lead distribution in rat organs corresponded to typical profiles and were in a good accordance with data published previously [37]. Risk assessments for toxicants in environmental media via oral exposure often rely on measurements of total concentration in a collected sample. However, the digestive system cannot mobilize all of a toxicant present in the binding matrix, and cannot absorb it with near 100% efficiency.

Although the higher doses of Pb caused its accumulation mainly in the gastrointestinal system (small and large intestine and stomach), indicating the growing inability of intestinal epithelial transport mechanisms to absorb Pb, we could show certain increases in the epitheliumal permeability induced by lead (II). This allows us to assume that default values of 30% lead bioavailability or somewhat even higher [51] might be a reasonable indicator for dosage.

The gastrointestinal microflora is a complex ecological system, normally characterized by a flexible equilibrium. Bifidobacteria and lactobacilli are Gram-positive lactic acid-producing bacteria constituting a major part of the intestinal microflora in humans and other mammals [52]. Successful probiotic bacteria are usually able to colonize the intestine, at least temporarily, by adhering to the intestinal mucosa. By doing that, probiotic bacteria might prevent the attachment of pathogens, such as coli-form bacteria and clostridia, and stimulate their removal from an infected intestinal tract.

Administration of antimicrobial agents notoriously causes disturbances in the ecological balance of the gastrointestinal microflora with several unwanted effects such as colonization by potential pathogens; many of them belonging to lactose-negative coli bacteria [53].

To our knowledge, our study in 2009 [40] was the first one to show a relation between dysbacteriosis and oral lead exposure.

Taking into account that different microbial groups have different susceptibilities to lead, population shifts in intestinal flora upon increasing Pb(II) concentrations were to be expected. Indeed, the CFU method showed clearly that the intake of lead (II) caused explosive growth of lactose-negative *E. coli* variants. In contrast, the yeasts, lactobacilli and lactose-positive coli bacteria were suppressed in proportion to lead concentration. Although particular health-related consequences of the shift in proportions of non-lactose fermenting relative to lactose-fermenting bacteria are not yet clear yet, rapid uncontrollable proliferation of lac(-) strains could be considered as an ecological imbalance causing a pathological state, referred to as dysbiosis or dysbacteriosis, which affects many aspects of gastrointestinal system function.

The most important role of the commensal microflora, from the point of view of the host, is to act in colonization resistance against exogenous, potentially pathogenic, microorganisms [54].

Thus, one of the causes of the observed lead-induced dysbacteriosis could be the disturbance in microbial adhesion to epithelia. To verify this hypothesis, a series of model *in-vitro* experiments can be performed. Recently, several laboratory models using human and rat intestinal cell lines have been developed to study the adhesion of bacteria [55].

Our *in vitro* study showesd clear differences in lead influence on adsorption profiles between Lac$^-$ (i^+ z^+ y^-) *E. coli* strain (representing a pathological group) and *Lactobacillus plantarum* ATCC 14917 (known as a probiotic strain).

In contrast to *Lactobacillus*, there was a broad range of lead concentrations where the adhesion of *E. coli* cells was not inhibited but rather stimulated as compared to the control. The particular molecular reasons for this phenomenon are unclear and could include both unspecific changes in electrostatic interactions and Pb-induced conformational rearrangements of surface proteins. The fact of Sstrong Pb interactions with proteins hasve been repeatedly confirmed in our laboratory and was were briefly presented in this chapter as the BSA aggregation phenomenon.

One of the principal difficulties in modeling intestinal environments lies in the uncertainty over mechanical stresses, molecular species involved as well as the topology and composition of the surfaces. The cultured cell model is a simple system that excludes many physiological variables such as peristalsis, blood flow, gastric emptying, etc., allowing the adsorption processes to be studied in isolation.

Nevertheless, there are obvious limitations with cell culture techniques, including the lack of systemic control, short incubation times, etc. Thus, we realize that in these studies the adhesion process only partially mimics the *in vivo* interactions of bacterial and intestinal cells and that the data must be interpreted guardedly.

To finalize, three concluding remarks can be formulated. First, the oral exposure of human beings and animals to *low* Pb concentrations deserves more careful attention. Lead doses that were much lower than those causing visible harmful effects on cell culture or on the level of the whole body could induce significant changes in intestinal microflora. The presence of Pb somehow creates selective advantages for pathological lactose-negative coli forms and thus contributes to dysbacteriosis development. Second, the adhesion of bacteria to intestinal epithelium is a possible cause of lead-induced dysbacteriosis. Third, the results could be possibly extrapolated to human beings, opening the opportunity of understanding some mysterious cases of persistent dysbacteriosis as a result of latent Pb intoxication. This, in turn, would suggest probiotic treatment as a promising therapy for lead-exposed patients on the one hand and the possibility of Pb-scavenging therapy for some patients with dysbacteriosis on the other. Regarding public health, monitoring and control over Pb intestinal levels would not only diminish the risk of lead specific pathologies, but would also be of major importance in maintaining the normal gut microflora.

Acknowledgments

The study was supported by PhD Program of Kazakh National University and members of the Institute for Bioengineering in Jülich, Germany.

References

[1] Heath, L. M., et al., Toxicity of environmental lead and the influence of intestinal absorption in children. *Rev. Environ. Health*, 2003. 18(4): p. 231-50.

[2] Ros, C. and L. Mwanri, Lead exposure, interactions and toxicity: food for thought. *Asia Pac. J. Clin. Nutr.*, 2003. 12(4): p. 388-95.

[3] Chang, L. W., The neurotoxicology and pathology of organomercury, organolead, and organotin. *J. Toxicol. Sci.*, 1990. 15 Suppl. 4: p. 125-51.

[4] Mudipalli, A., Lead hepatotoxicity and potential health effects. *Indian J. Med. Res*., 2007. 126(6): p. 518-27.

[5] Bogden, J. D., J. M. Oleske and D. B. Louria, Lead poisoning--one approach to a problem that won't go away. *Environ. Health Perspect.*, 1997. 105(12): p. 1284-7.

[6] Maas, R. P., et al., Reducing lead exposure from drinking water: recent history and current status. *Public Health Rep.*, 2005. 120(3): p. 316-21.

[7] Firestone, M., et al., Potential new approaches for children's inhalation risk assessment. *J. Toxicol. Environ. Health A*, 2008. 71(3): p. 208-17.

[8] Flury, F. and F. Zernik, *Zusammenstellung der toxischen und letalen Dosen für die gebräuchlichsten Gifte und Versuchstiere*. 1928: Urban and Schwarzenberg.
[9] Cunningham, G., Lead--toxicology and assessment in general practice. *Aust. Fam. Physician*, 2007. 36(12): p. 1011-3.
[10] Lukacs, A., et al., Subchronic heavy metal and alcohol treatment in rats: changes in the somatosensory evoked cortical activity. *Acta Biol. Hung.*, 2007. 58(3): p. 259-67.
[11] Sharma, V. K., et al., Organic-coated silver nanoparticles in biological and environmental conditions: fate, stability and toxicity. *Adv. Colloid Interface Sci.*, 2014. 204: p. 15-34.
[12] Tahiri, M., et al., The rhamnogalacturonan-II dimer decreases intestinal absorption and tissue accumulation of lead in rats. *J. Nutr.*, 2000. 130(2): p. 249-53.
[13] Beak, D. G., et al., Bioaccessibility of lead sequestered to corundum and ferrihydrite in a simulated gastrointestinal system. *J. Environ. Qual.*, 2006. 35(6): p. 2075-83.
[14] Breton, J., et al., Chronic ingestion of cadmium and lead alters the bioavailability of essential and heavy metals, gene expression pathways and genotoxicity in mouse intestine. *Arch. Toxicol.*, 2013. 87(10): p. 1787-95.
[15] Cerklewski, F. L. and R. M. Forbes, Influence of dietary zinc on lead toxicity in the rat. *J. Nutr.*, 1976. 106(5): p. 689-96.
[16] Fullmer, C. S., Lead-calcium interactions: involvement of 1,25-dihydroxy vitamin D. *Environ. Res.*, 1997. 72(1): p. 45-55.
[17] Wise, A., Protective action of calcium phytate against acute lead toxicity in mice. *Bull. Environ. Contam. Toxicol.*, 1981. 27(5): p. 630-3.
[18] Conrad, M. E. and J. C. Barton, Factors affecting the absorption and excretion of lead in the rat. *Gastroenterology*, 1978. 74(4): p. 731-40.
[19] Verschoyle, R. D. and R. A. Little, The acute toxicity of some organolead and organotin compounds in the rat, with particular reference to a gastric lesion. *J. Appl. Toxicol.*, 1981. 1(5): p. 247-55.
[20] Finkelstein, Y., M. E. Markowitz and J. F. Rosen, Low-level lead-induced neurotoxicity in children: an update on central nervous system effects. *Brain Res. Brain Res. Rev.*, 1998. 27(2): p. 168-76.
[21] D'Argenio, V. and F. Salvatore, The role of the gut microbiome in the healthy adult status. *Clin. Chim. Acta*, 2015.
[22] Savino, F., et al., Intestinal microflora in breastfed colicky and non-colicky infants. *Acta Paediatr.*, 2004. 93(6): p. 825-9.

[23] Sun, J. and E. B. Chang, Exploring gut microbes in human health and disease: Pushing the envelope. *Genes Dis.*, 2014. 1(2): p. 132-139.
[24] Nielsen, O. H., New strategies for treatment of inflammatory bowel disease. *Front. Med.* (Lausanne), 2014. 1: p. 3.
[25] Morawiec, M., [Effects of harmful trace elements on iron, zinc and copper: their interactions in animals and humans. II. Lead]. *Rocz. Panstw Zakl. Hig.*, 1991. 42(2): p. 121-6.
[26] Company, A. C., *Classes of Compounds and Numerical Cross Reference List.* 1990: Aldrich Chemical Company.
[27] Couto, M., Laboratory guidelines for animal care. *Methods Mol. Biol.*, 2011. 770: p. 579-99.
[28] Yee, H. Y., J. D. Nelson and B. Jackson, Measurement of lead in blood by graphite furnace atomic absorption spectrometry. *J. Anal. Toxicol.*, 1994. 18(7): p. 415-8.
[29] Iturri, S. J. and A. Pena, Heavy metal-induced inhibition of active transport in the rat small intestine in vitro. Interaction with other ions. *Comp. Biochem. Physiol. C*, 1986. 84(2): p. 363-8.
[30] Tomczok, J., et al., Ultrastructural aspects of the small intestinal lead toxicology. Part I: Surface ultrastructure of the small intestine mucosa in rats with lead acetate poisoning. *Exp. Pathol.*, 1988. 35(1): p. 49-55.
[31] Tomczok, J., et al., Ultrastructural aspects of the small intestinal lead toxicology. Part II. The small intestine goblet cells of rats during lead poisoning. *Exp. Pathol.*, 1988. 35(2): p. 93-100.
[32] Quaroni, A., et al., Epithelioid cell cultures from rat small intestine. Characterization by morphologic and immunologic criteria. *J. Cell Biol.*, 1979. 80(2): p. 248-65.
[33] Lee, Y. K., et al., Quantitative approach in the study of adhesion of lactic acid bacteria to intestinal cells and their competition with enterobacteria. *Appl. Environ. Microbiol.*, 2000. 66(9): p. 3692-7.
[34] Demirci, E. K., et al., rhAPC reduces the endothelial cell permeability via a decrease of contractile tensions induced by endothelial cells. *J. Biosci. Bioeng.*, 2012. 114(2): p. 212-9.
[35] Arosio, D., et al., Static and dynamic light scattering approach to the hydration of hemoglobin and its supertetramers in the presence of osmolites. *Biopolymers*, 2002. 63(1): p. 1-11.
[36] Digel, I., et al., Body temperature-related structural transitions of monotremal and human hemoglobin. *Biophys. J.*, 2006. 91(8): p. 3014-21.

[37] Kostial, K., I. Simonovic and M. Pisonic, Lead absorption from the intestine in newborn rats. *Nature*, 1971. 233(5321): p. 564.

[38] Struzynska, L., et al., Lead-induced abnormalities in blood-brain barrier permeability in experimental chronic toxicity. *Mol. Chem. Neuropathol.*, 1997. 31(3): p. 207-24.

[39] Jacob, F. and J. Monod, Genetic regulatory mechanisms in the synthesis of proteins. *J. Mol. Biol.*, 1961. 3: p. 318-56.

[40] Sadykov, R., et al., Oral lead exposure induces dysbacteriosis in rats. *J. Occup. Health*, 2009. 51(1): p. 64-73.

[41] Tamas, M. J., et al., Heavy metals and metalloids as a cause for protein misfolding and aggregation. *Biomolecules*, 2014. 4(1): p. 252-67.

[42] White, L. D., et al., New and evolving concepts in the neurotoxicology of lead. *Toxicol. Appl. Pharmacol.*, 2007. 225(1): p. 1-27.

[43] Sekimoto, Y., et al., Removal of Pb(II) from water using keratin colloidal solution obtained from wool. *Environ. Sci. Pollut. Res. Int.*, 2013. 20(9): p. 6531-8.

[44] Bassam, R., et al., Effects of spermine NONOate and ATP on protein aggregation: light scattering evidences. *BMC Biophys.*, 2013. 6: p. 1.

[45] Chen, M., et al., Structural changes of human serum albumin induced by cadmium acetate. *J. Biochem. Mol. Toxicol.*, 2014. 28(6): p. 281-7.

[46] Lu, Y., et al., Assessment of bioaccessibility and exposure risk of arsenic and lead in urban soils of Guangzhou City, China. *Environ. Geochem. Health*, 2011. 33(2): p. 93-102.

[47] Darshan, D., D. M. Fraze and G. J. Anderson, Molecular basis of iron-loading disorders. *Expert Rev. Mol. Med.*, 2010. 12: p. e36.

[48] Fullmer, C. S. and J. F. Rosen, Effect of dietary calcium and lead status on intestinal calcium absorption. *Environ. Res.*, 1990. 51(1): p. 91-9.

[49] Marchetti, C., I. Baranowska-Bosiacka and P. Gavazzo, Multiple effects of copper on NMDA receptor currents. *Brain Res.*, 2014. 1542: p. 20-31.

[50] Othman, M., R. Aguero and H. C. Lin, Alterations in intestinal microbial flora and human disease. *Curr. Opin. Gastroenterol.*, 2008. 24(1): p. 11-6.

[51] Yu, C. H., L. M. Yiin and P. J. Lioy, The bioaccessibility of lead (Pb) from vacuumed house dust on carpets in urban residences. *Risk Anal.*, 2006. 26(1): p. 125-34.

[52] Fukuda, S. and H. Ohno, Gut microbiome and metabolic diseases. *Semin. Immunopathol.*, 2014. 36(1): p. 103-14.

[53] Salonen, A., W. M. de Vos and A. Palva, Gastrointestinal microbiota in irritable bowel syndrome: present state and perspectives. *Microbiology*, 2010. 156(Pt 11): p. 3205-15.
[54] Ouwehand, A. C., P. Niemi and S. J. Salminen, The normal faecal microflora does not affect the adhesion of probiotic bacteria in vitro. *FEMS Microbiol. Lett.*, 1999. 177(1): p. 35-8.
[55] Greene, J. D. and T. R. Klaenhammer, Factors involved in adherence of lactobacilli to human Caco-2 cells. *Appl. Environ. Microbiol.*, 1994. 60 (12): p. 4487-94.

In: Lead Exposure and Poisoning
Editor: Leonard Horton
ISBN: 978-1-63482-699-0

Chapter IV

Fractions of Sarcocornia Perennis Extract Protect Human Kidney Cells against Lead Induced Oxidative Stress and Apoptosis

Manel Gargouri[1,2, 3,4], Hélène Talarmin[2], Riadh Ksouri[3], Marie-Agnès Giroux Metges[2] and Christian Magné[4,*]

[1]Laboratoire d'Ecophysiologie Animale,
Faculté des Sciences de Sfax, Sfax, Tunisia
[2]EA 1274, Faculté de Médecine et Sciences de la Santé, Université de Bretagne Occidentale, Brest Cedex, France
[3]Laboratoire des Plantes Extrêmophiles,
Centre de Biotechnologie de Borj-Cedria, Tunisia
[4]EA 2219 Géoarchitecture, UFR Sciences et Techniques,
Université de Bretagne Occidentale, Brest Cedex, France

[*] Corresponding author: Christian MAGNE, Phone: +33 298 01 6247, Fax: +33 298 01 6721, E-mail: christian.magne@univ-brest.fr.

Abstract

Lead (Pb) exposure is known to induce a wide range of physiological and biochemical dysfunctions in humans and animals. We previously showed that lead causes oxidative damage and cytotoxicity in human kidney cells. Now, we report the effects of fractions of the edible halophyte *Sarcocornia perennis* on these cells after Pb intoxication. HEK 293 cells were seeded in 96-well plates in medium containing Pb with or without fractions of *S. perennis* methanolic extract. Morphological and biochemical indicators were used to evaluate cytoprotective and antioxidant effects of the extract fractions.

Our results showed that lead induced (1) a decrease in cell viability, (2) apoptosis, (3) cell distortion and cohesion loss, and (4) superoxide anion production and lipid peroxidation. These observations were alleviated upon addition of $MeOH_{80}$ fraction of plant extract and, to a lower extent, $MeOH_{60}$ one. Our results suggest that *S. perennis* contains promisful substances to counteract the lead intoxication.

Keywords: cytotoxicity, extract fractionation, kidney cells, lead, oxidative stress, perennial glasswort

Abbreviations

DMEM	Dulbecco's modified Eagle's medium;
DMSO	Dimethyl sulfoxide;
EDTA	Ethylene diamine tetraacetic acid;
FBS	Fetal bovine serum;
HEK	Human embryonic kidney;
MDA	Malondialdehyde;
MTT	3-(4,5-dimethylthiazol-2-yl)-2,5-diphenyl tetrazolium bromide;
NBT	Nitroblue tetrazolium;
PBS	Phosphate buffer saline;
PMSF	Phenylmethanesulfonyl fluoride;
ROS	Reactive oxygen species;
TBA	Thiobarbituric acid;
TBARS	Thiobarbituric acid reactive substances;
TCA	Trichloroacetic acid;
Tris	1,1,1- (trihydroxylmethyl) ethane.

1. Introduction

With the worldwide increase of industrial pollution and manmade or natural combustion activities, we are all exposed either voluntarily or not to certain environmental pollutants such as heavy metals, organic hydrocarbons, and pesticides, from various sources. Lead (Pb) is one of the most widely used metals in industries and in many countries exposure to Pb continues to be a widespread problem (Xiang et al., 2010). This metal is also known to induce a wide range of physiological, biochemical and behavioral dysfunctions both in animals and human beings (Needleman, 2004). Pb is a non-threshold multi-targeted toxicant that causes alterations in different organs of the body, including the kidney (Lin et al., 2001; Jarrar 2003; Navarro-Moreno et al., 2009; Abdel-Moneim et al., 2011). Kidney plays a critical role in the uptake, metabolism and elimination of numerous drugs and other chemicals. It possesses some unique physiology and metabolic pathways (Lohr et al., 1998). As a consequence of this and because of the presence of certain enzymatic pathways within the kidneys, many chemicals may exert renal selective toxicity. Numerous in vitro models, most of them using tissues from laboratory animals such as the rat, have been developed to study mechanisms of renal injury induced by environmental chemicals and other xenobiotics. Although the precise mechanism of kidney toxicity caused by Pb is not clear, there is evidence that Pb can cause generation of reactive oxygen metabolites and inhibits the activity of antioxidant enzymes in kidney tissue (Pulido and Parrish 2003; Jurczuk et al., 2007; Franco et al., 2009; Abdel-Moneim et al., 2011). Recent studies also indicated that Pb can induce DNA injury in kidney and these effects were shown to be associated with ROS formation resulting in caspase-3 dependent apoptosis (Liu et al., 2010). As inactive dimers, the caspase-3 zymogens pre-exist within the cytosol (Boatright et al., 2003). They are activated through limited proteolysis within their interdomain linker by an initiator caspases, and occasionally by other proteases under specific circumstances (Salvesen and Abrams, 2004). In multiple cell types, activated caspase-3 will result in certain apoptotic hallmarks, such as chromatin condensation and DNA fragmentation (Woo et al., 1998). Therefore, the topic of lead induced apoptosis need further study. Due to the intrinsic limitations and variability of efficacy of heavy metal chelating agents, Pb intoxication therapy is looking for the development of new therapeutic agents with different modes of action especially from (the) medicinal plants. In recent years, the clinical importance of herbal drugs has received considerable attention. As many synthetic antioxidants have been shown to have one or the other side effects (Nocentini et al., 2001) there has been an upsurge of interest in the therapeutic potential of medicinal plants as antioxidants in reducing free radical-induced tissue injury (Koleva et al., 2002). Although salt marsh plants were recognized environmentally as one of the most important ecosystems in a tidal zone because they play vital roles in the tidal ecology, such as serving as buffers, protecting the shorelines from erosion by the force of waves, and filtering contaminants from the land, their biological activities as well as their secondary metabolites have been little reported until now (Bang et al., 2002; Jo et al., 2002; Han et al., 2003). In this context, Sarcocornia genera, from the family Chenopodiaceae, contains edible species (Heller 1953) which produces succulent shoots suitable for leafy vegetable production, and has been recently characterized in terms of yield and nutritional value (Ventura et al., 2011). A Sarcocornia plant, which is a perennial herb, has been introduced into the European market as a vegetable with leafless shoots resembling green asparagus. The young fleshy tips of this green vegetable are in high demand in gourmet kitchens, not only for their salty taste, but also for their high nutritional content, which includes proteins, carbohydrates, fiber, calcium, potassium, magnesium, iron, manganese, copper, beta-carotene and antioxidant vitamins such as vitamin C which made it an ideal diet supplement (Lu et al., 2001). In particular, a Sarcocornia enriched product with nutritionally valuable metabolites, such as omega-3 fatty acids, phenolic compounds, antioxidants or minerals is thought to meet the standards of „functional food" for health enthusiast (Del Giudice and Pascucci 2010). Therefore, as a part of our first attempt of analyses for new antioxidants compounds from natural sources (Lee et al., 2004; Park et al., 2004; Seo et al., 2004), we tried to screen the effect of halophyte extract (*S. perennis*), recognized as new sources, on oxidative damage caused by lead intoxication in human kidney cells.

2. Materials and Methods

2.1. Chemicals

Dulbecco's modified Eagle's medium (DMEM), fetal bovine serum (FBS), phosphate buffer saline (PBS), antibiotic mixture (penicillin + streptomycin) and trypan blue solution were purchased from Lonza (Cologne Gmbh,

Germany). Lead acetate was purchased from Merck KGaA (Frankfurter, Germany). Other chemicals were purchased from Sigma Chemicals Co. (St. Louis, MO, USA).

2.2. Biological

2.2.1. Plant Material

Sarcocornia perennis L. (= *Salicornia perennis L, Arthrocnemum perenne L*), also known as perennial glasswort, is a succulent saltbush native from Atlantic and Mediterranean shorelines. Plants were collected in September 2009 at Korba in Tunisia. One sample was recorded in the herbarium at the Biotechnology Centre of Borj-Cedria (ASP-72). The plant material was frozen and subsequently freeze-dried prior to use.

2.2.2. Cell Line and Culture

Human embryonic kidney (HEK) 293 cell line was purchased from American Type Culture Collection (ATTC, CRL-1573). Cells were grown in DMEM supplemented with 10% FBS and antibiotics (100 UI mL^{-1} penicillin G and 100 μg mL^{-1} streptomycin). The cell culture was incubated at 37°C in a humidified atmosphere containing 5% CO_2/ 95% air.

The viability of the cells was assessed by trypan blue (0.4%, w/v) exclusion prior to start each experiment. The batches showing more that 95% cell viability were used in the study.

2.3. Preparation of Different Fractions Extracts and Lead Solutions

2.3.1. Extraction, Clean up and Fractionation

The powder (10 g) of each organ was extracted three times by 50 mL hexane to remove lipids and pigments. The resulting residue was re-suspended in 100 mL methanol 80 (three times). Each extraction was carried out by maceration in the solvent for 5 min under magnetic stirring, and the mixture was filtered through a Whatmann N°4 filter paper. Methanol filtrates were combined, concentrated under vacuum using a rotary evaporator at 40°C and fractionated on reverse phase silica gel (Guyot et al., 1998). One mL of methanolic extracts was loaded onto the column containing 10 g of C18 resin

(Silica gel 100 C18, 0.040-0.063 mm, 230-400 mesh ASTM – Fluka ®). The different compounds adsorbed onto the resin were then eluted with 20 mL of increasing MeOH concentrations (successively 20, 40, 50, 60, 80 and 100% methanol in water). The obtained fractions were separately evaporated to dryness, weighed to obtain the dry residue and solubilized in 1 mL of deuterated solvent (D_2O or MeOD) to conduct NMR analyses. Alternatively, a 10 μL aliquot of extract was diluted in DMEM to a final methanol concentration of 0.025% for toxicological studies.

2.3.2. Preparation of Lead Solutions

A 30 mM stock solution of Pb (acetate form) was prepared in H_2O. Then, that solution was diluted in DMEM at final Pb concentrations ranging from 0 to 1600 μM.

2.4. Renal Cell Treatments

HEK 293 cells were seeded in 96-well plates (4 x 10^4 cells $well^{-1}$ in 200 μL medium) and allowed to adhere for 24 h at 37°C in a 5% CO_2/95% air incubator. Medium was aspirated and replaced with medium containing Pb ranging from 50 to 1600 μM with or without different fractions of *Sarcocornia*. Some cultures were also incubated with only the vehicle solvent (0.025% methanol). Experiments were realized at least three times and tested in six separate wells for each condition.

2.5. Analysis of Cell Parameters

2.5.1. Morphology

In order to evaluate morphological modifications in the presence of Pb with or without non-toxic fractions of *Sarcocornia*, cells were observed with inverted microscope (Olympus optical CO-LTD, BH_2-RFL-T_3) after 24 h of treatment.

2.5.2. Cell Viability

Cell viability was determined by the MTT method (Upreti et al., 2007). After cell treatment, 0.5 mg mL^{-1} MTT was added to each well and plates were incubated for 2 h at 37°C. In viable cells, MTT is converted to purple formazan dye, which is measured spectrophotometrically (Bio-Teck Instruments) at 540 nm after solubilization in 100 μL of DMSO.

2.5.3. Caspase-3 Enzymatic Activity Assay

Caspase 3/7 activity was measured using the caspase- glo ®3/7 assay kit (Promega) in HEK 293 cells treated with Pb (from 50 to 1600 μM) with or without fractions of *Sarcocornia* for 24 h. Briefly, the pro-luminescent substrate containing the tetrapeptide DEVD was cleaved by caspase, which resulted in the release of aminoluciferin (a substrate for luciferase). After reaction with luciferase, luminescent signal was produced and measured with a luminometer (MLX Microtiter Plate Luminometer, Dynex). The positive control of apoptosis was induced by 200 μM of H_2O_2.

2.5.4. Superoxide Anion Production

The superoxide anion produced by renal cells upon treatments was assessed using the nitroblue tetrazolium (NBT) assay, which measures the conversion of NBT to blue formazan (Pick 1986). After each treatment, cells were incubated with 0.5 mg mL^{-1} NBT in culture medium for 2 h at 37°C. Produced formazan was determined spectrophotometrically at 560 nm after solubilization in 100 μL of DMSO.

2.5.5. Lipid Peroxidation

Lipid peroxidation products were quantified by measuring TBARS by the method of Yagi (Yagi 1976). HEK 293 cells were seeded in an amount of 10^6 cells in 25 cm^2 tissue flasks and grown in DMEM supplemented with 10% FBS and antibiotics (100 UI mL^{-1} penicillin G and 100 μg mL^{-1} streptomycin) in a humidified atmosphere of 5% CO_2 at 37°C. The cells were treated for 24 h with Pb (50, 500, 800 and 1600 μM) with or without plant extract. The cells were washed with ice cold PBS, detached and sonicated at 4°C in 500 μL of lysis buffer (Tris/HCl 0.1 M, pH 7.4). After homogenization, the mixture was centrifuged (13000 *g* for 10 min at 4°C) and protein concentration was determined in the supernatant using Bradford method (1976). Then, 125 μL of supernatant were mixed with 125 μL of TCA in order to discard proteins and after centrifugation (1000 *g*, 10 min, 4°C), 200 μL of the new supernatant were mixed with 40 μL HCl (0.6 M) and 160 μL of thiobarbituric acid (TBA) 20% in TBS. The mixture was heated at 80°C for 10 min and, after cooling to room temperature, the absorbance was read at 530 nm using the molar extinction coefficient of the MDA-TBA complex (1.56×10^5 $M^{-1}cm^{-1}$).

2.6. Data Analysis and Statistics

Experiments were carried out at least three times and the data presented are the mean ± SE from independent experiments. Comparisons were made with appropriate controls employing Student *t* test. Differences were considered significant at different levels ($P < 0.05$; $P < 0.01$; $P < 0.001$).

3. Results and Discussion

Extracts of *Sarcocornia perennis* were fractionated through a C_{18} column into 6 fractions, eluted successively with 20, 40, 50, 60, 80 and 100% methanol solutions. Since the 20% methanol fraction did not contain enough materials for further experiments, the other five fractions were tested on human kidney cells (HEK 293, non-tumor cells). The effect of *S. perennis* fractions on cell viability was presented in figure 1. Methanol alone until 0.5% (v/v) did not affect the viability of the cultures after 24 h of exposure (data not shown). Among the 5 fractions of plant extract, two ($MeOH_{60}$ and $MeOH_{80}$) did not show any toxicity on HEK 293 cells. Conversely, $MeOH_{40}$ fraction caused 20% mortality and the last two fractions ($MeOH_{50}$ and $MeOH_{100}$) induced 30% loss of viability, suggesting that these fractions contain toxic components. Literature on the potent role of halophytic plant extract in cell protection is scarce. Only Seo et al., (2005) showed that some salt marsh species, including *Rosa rugosa*, *Ixeris tamagawaensis*, *Artemisia capillaris*, *Tetragonia tetragonoides*, *Erigeron annuus* and *Glehnia littoralis* may maintain cell proliferation while others are inefficient in suppressing cell death. Also, in a previous work, we showed that *S. perennis* raw extract was able to partially restore cell viability upon lead intoxication (Gargouri et al., 2013).

Then, for the first time, we fractioned raw extract from that perennial plant to determine which fraction was active *in vitro* on cells exposed to lead. Present results showed that 60% MeOH fraction improves the viability of kidney cells treated with lead (up to 800 μM) (Figure 2.A). Noteworthy was the total recovery of cell viability with 80% MeOH fraction at any Pb concentration (Figure 2.B). That fraction also thwarted the cell deformation (loss of cohesion, rounding) induced by lead (Figure 3.C, 3.D, 3.E and 3.F) and restored normal morphology (Figure 3.C', 3.D', 3.E' and 3.F'). Our results are in agreement with other *in vitro* studies indicating that seaweeds exert stimulatory activities on human cell proliferation (Liu et al., 1997; Shan et al., 1999).

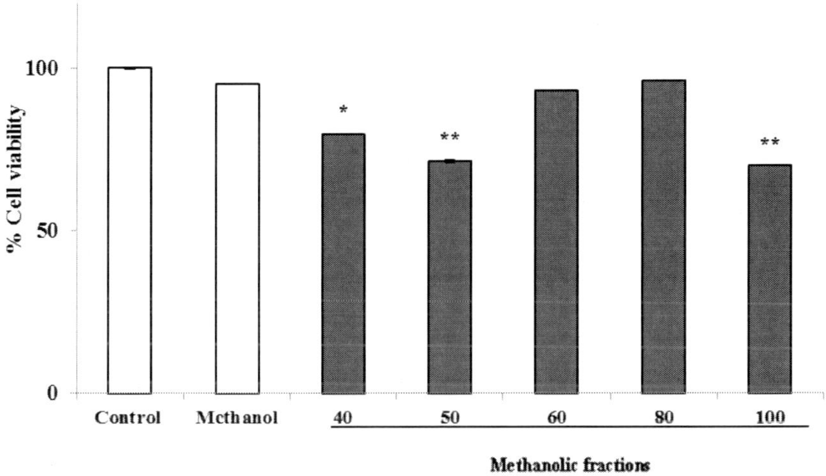

Figure 1. Cell viability measured by MTT assay in HEK 293 cells after 24 h of treatment with different fractions of *Sarcocornia perennis*. The values are expressed by mean ± SEM of three independent experiments. Number of determinations for each column: n = 6 Significant differences between groups were mentioned as follows: Methanolic fractions (40%, 50%, 60%, 80% and 100%) group compared to control: *P < 0.05; **P < 0.01.

All the above mentioned morphological changes caused by Pb treatment in HEK-293 cells could be explained by the induction of apoptosis process. On that point, recent studies indicated that apoptosis is associated with the lead-induced cytotoxicity (Pulido and Parrish 2003; Liu et al., 2010). Accordingly, cells exposed to lead for 24 hours exhibited an increased caspase activity, in a dose-dependent manner (Figure 4). A 2-fold induction of enzyme activity was found under 1600 μM Pb (P<0.001), thereby leading to apoptosis since caspases are well-known mediators of cell death (Fan et al., 2005). Conversely, cells treated with 80% MeOH fraction of *Sarcocornia perennis* extract concomitantly with Pb (up to 500 μM) did not undergo apoptosis, as shown by the decrease of the caspase-3 activity (Figure 4). This suggested that plant extract protects kidney cell by reversing the Pb toxicity. At higher lead concentrations, however, the methanol fraction, although inhibiting significantly caspase 3 activity (P<0.001), did not restore control level.

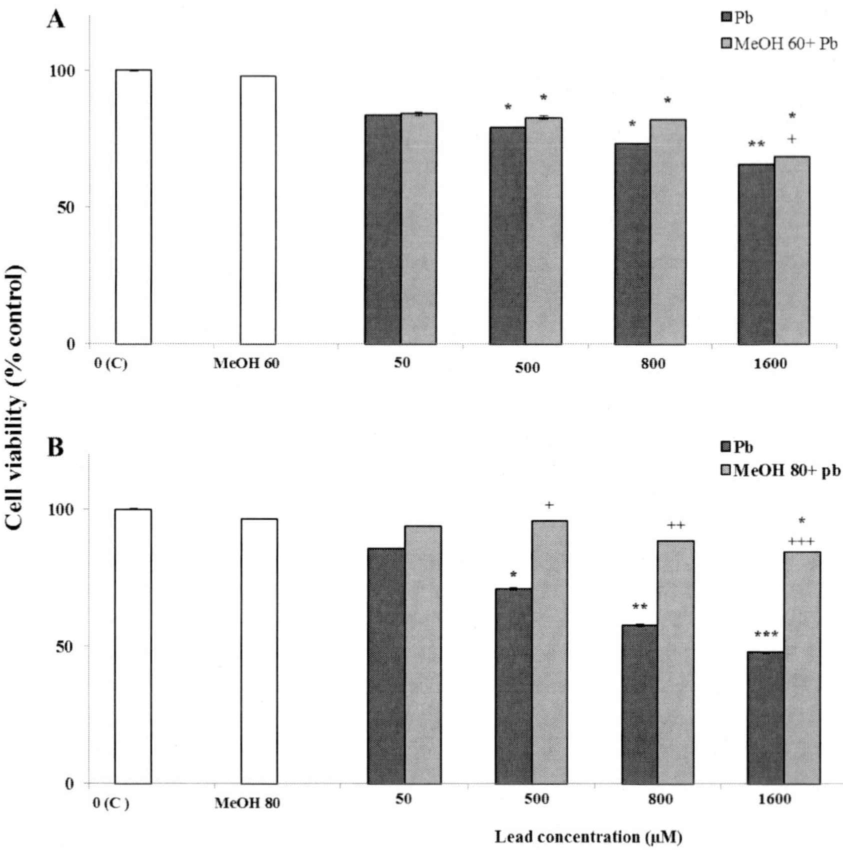

Figure 2. HEK 293 cell viability following a 24 h exposure to Pb alone or with $MeOH_{60}$ fraction (Fig. 2A) or $MeOH_{80}$ (Figure 2B). The values are expressed by mean ± SEM of three independent experiments Number of determinations for each column: n = 6. Significant differences between groups were mentioned as follows:*: Comparison of Pb (50, 500, 800 or 1600 µM) to control. +: Comparison of $MeOH_{60}$ fraction + Pb (50, 500, 800 or 1600 µM) to lead (Pb). One symbol: $P < 0.05$; Two symbols: $P < 0.01$; Three symbols: $P < 0.001$.

While lead toxicity is associated with an apoptosis-like form of cell death (Madden et al., 2002; Xu et al., 2006), it has also been reported to trigger the production of reactive oxygen species (Franco et al., 2009; Liu et al., 2010; Gargouri et al., 2013). Accordingly, our results showed that lead acetate induces $O_2^{\cdot-}$ production in HEK 293 cells by 22%, 34%, 45% and 63% in the presence of 50, 500, 800 and 1600 µM Pb, respectively (Figure 5). Moreover, we found that Pb caused an increase in the levels of TBARS, a stable lipid peroxidation marker (Girotti et al., 1991; Marnett 2002), in a dose-dependent manner (Figure 6).

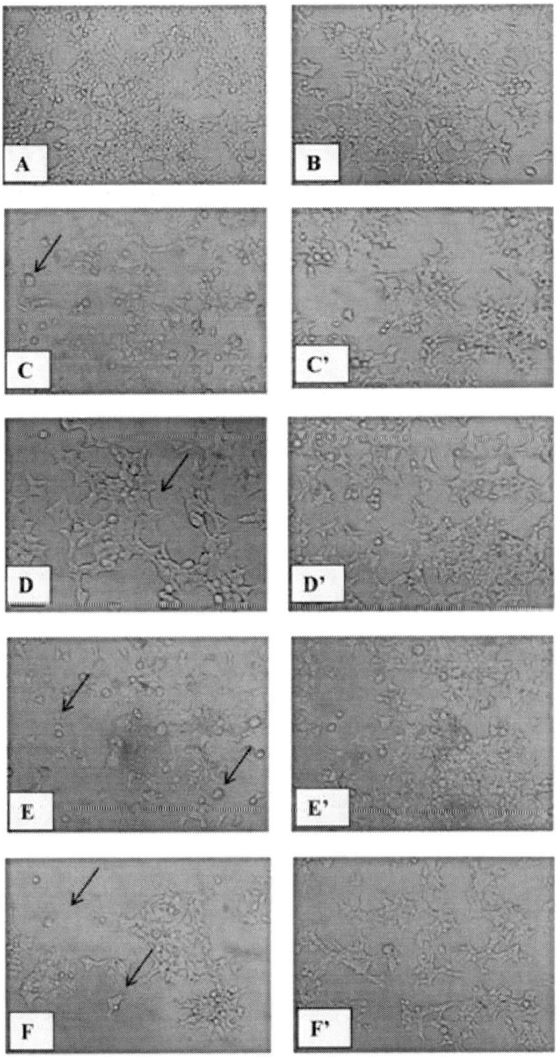

→ Deformation (or lysis) of cells induced by Pb.

Figure 3. Pb affected morphology of HEK 293 cells. The morphology of HEK 293 cells after exposure to the different doses of Pb alone or concomitantly with fraction MeOH80 for 24 h was examined by contrast microscopy (100 x). (3A) Control; (3B) Methanol; (3C) 50 μM Pb; (3D) 500 μM Pb; (3E) 800 μM Pb; (3F) 1600 μM Pb; (3C') 50 μM Pb+ MeOH80; (3D') 500 μM Pb+ MeOH80; (3E') 800 μM Pb+ MeOH80; (3F') 1600 μM Pb+ MeOH80.

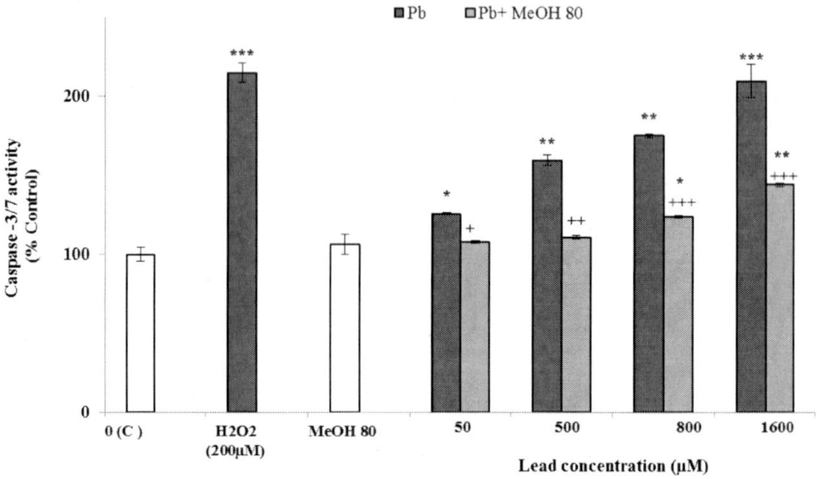

Figure 4. Activity of caspase 3/7 in HEK 293 cells after 24 h exposure to Pb alone or with MeOH 80 fraction. The values are expressed by mean ± SEM of one independent experiment. Number of determinations for each column: n = 3. Significant differences between groups were mentioned as follows: *: Comparison of Pb (50, 500, 800 or 1600 µM) to control. +: Comparison of $MeOH_{80}$ + Pb (50, 500, 800 or 1600 µM) to lead (Pb). One symbol: $P < 0.05$; Two symbols: $P < 0.01$; Three symbols: $P < 0.001$.

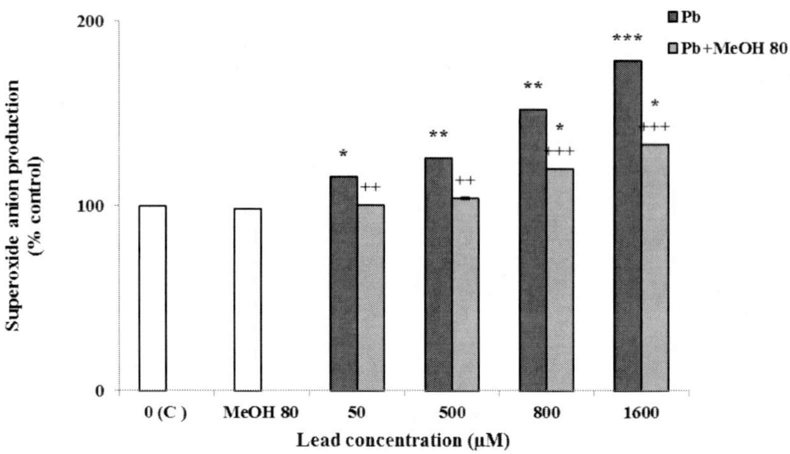

Figure 5. Measurement of superoxide anion production using NBT assay in HEK 293 cells following 24 h exposure to different concentrations of Pb alone or with $MeOH_{80}$. The values are expressed by mean ± SEM of three independent experiments. Number of determinations for each column: n = 6. Significant differences between groups were mentioned as follows: *: Comparison of Pb (50, 500, 800 or 1600 µM) to control. +: Comparison of $MeOH_{80}$ + Pb (50, 500, 800 or 1600 µM) to Pb. One symbol: $P < 0.05$; Two symbols: $P < 0.01$; Three symbols: $P < 0.001$.

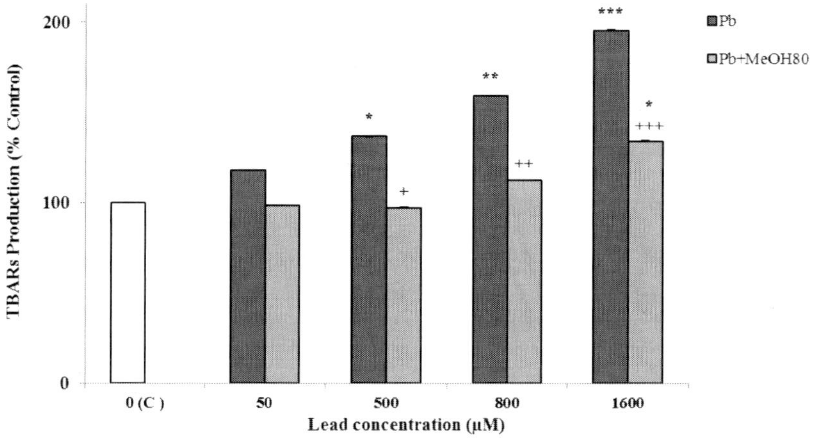

Figure 6. Lipid peroxidation in HEK 293 cells after 24h of treatment with Pb alone or with MeOH80 fraction. Number of determinations for each column: n = 4. Values are expressed as means ± SD. Significant differences between groups were mentioned as follows: *: Comparison of Pb (50, 500, 800 or 1600 µM) to control. +: Comparison of $MeOH_{80}$ + Pb (50, 500, 800 or 1600 µM) to Pb. One symbol: $P < 0.05$; Two symbols: $P < 0.01$; Three symbols: $P < 0.001$.

Conversely, the addition of $MeOH_{80}$ fraction induced a strong inhibition of superoxyde anion production and of lipid peroxidation compared to cells treated with Pb alone (Figure 6). In the presence of plant fraction, control oxidative status was recovered under 50 and 500 µM lead. Such protective action of plant extract against oxidative damage is likely related to its composition. Accordingly, 80% MeOH has often been used to extract phenolic compounds, which are known to possess antioxidant properties (Rice-Evans et al., 1997; Grace 2005). NMR analyses are under progress to elucidate the nature of active compounds present in that $MeOH_{80}$ fraction of *S. perennis* extract.

To our knowledge, this is the first report on the *in vitro* effects of plant fractions on the viability of intoxicated cells. Our results suggest that some salt marsh plants like *Sarcocornia perennis* could be valuable sources to treat or prevent oxidative damages. Further studies are in progress to investigate the composition and antioxidant properties of *S. perennis* fractions, in particular the active $MeOH_{60}$ and $MeOH_{80}$ ones, with the aim at isolating the bioactive compounds responsible for cell protection.

Acknowledgments

The authors acknowledge the receipt of a STSM grant to M.G. from the Agence Universitaire de la Francophonie.

References

Abdel-Moneim, AE; Dkhil, MA; Al-Quraishy, S. The potential role of flaxseed oil on lead acetate-induced kidney injury in adult male albino rats. *African Journal of Biotechnology*, 2011, 10, 1436-1451.

Bang, MA; Kim, HA; Kim, YJ. Hypoglycemic and antioxidant effect of dietary hamcho powder in streptozotocin induced diabetic rats. *Journal of Korean Society for Food Science and Nutrition*, 2002, 31, 840-846.

Boatright, KM; Renatus, M; Scott, FL; Sperandio, S; Shin, H; Pedersen, IM; Ricci, JE; Edris, WA; Sutherlin, DP; Green, DR; Salvesen, GS. A unified model for apical caspase activation. *Molecular Cell*, 2003, 11, 529-541.

Bradford, MM. A rapid and sensitive method for the quantitation of microgram quantities of protein utilizing the principle of protein-dye binding. *Analytical Biochemistry*, 1976, 72, 248-254.

Del Giudice, T; Pascucci, S. The role of consumer acceptance in the food innovation process: Young consumer perception of functional foods in Italy. *International Journal on Food System Dynamics*, 2010, 2, 111-122.

Fan, TJ; Han, LH; Cong, RS; Liang, J. Caspase family proteases and apoptosis. *Acta Biochimica et Biophysica Sinica*, 2005, 37, 719-727.

Franco, R; Sánchez-Olea, R; Reyes-Reyes, EM; Panayiotidis, MI. Environmental toxicity, oxidative stress and apoptosis: Ménage à Trois. *Mutation Research*, 2009, 674, 3-22.

Gargouri, M ; Magné, C; Dauvergne, X; Ksouri, R; El Feki, A; Giroux Metges, MA; Talarmin, H. Cytoprotective and antioxidant effects of the edible halophyte *Sarcocornia perennis* L. (swampfire) against lead-induced toxicity in renal cells. *Ecotoxicology and Environmental Safety*, 2013, 95, 44-51.

Girotti, MJ; Khan, N; McLellan, BA. Early measurement of systemic lipid peroxidation products in the plasma of major blunt trauma patients. *Journal of Trauma and Acute Care Surgery*, 1991. 31, 32-35.

Grace, SC. Phenolics and antioxidants. In: Smirnoff, N. (Ed.). Antioxidants and reactive oxygen species in plants. *Blackwell Publishing: Ltd*, 2005; 141-168.

Guyot, S; Marnet, N; Sanoner, P; Drilleau, JF. Direct thiolysis on crude apple materials for HPLC characterization and quantification of polyphenols in cider apple tissues and juices. *Methods in Enzymology*, 2001, 335, 57-70.

Han, SK; Kim, SM; Pyo, BS. Antioxidative effect of glasswort (*Salicornia herbacea* L.) on the lipid oxidation of pork. *Korean Journal for Food Science of Animal Resources*, 2003, 23, 46-49.

Heller, CA. Edible and poisonous plants. Ph.D. Thesis, University of Alaska; 1953.

Jarrar, BM. Histological and histochemical alterations in the kidney induced by lead. *Annals of Saudi Medicine*, 2003, 23, 10-15.

Jo, YC; Ahn, JH; Chon, SM; Lee, KS; Bae, TJ; Kang, DS. Studies on pharmacological effects of glasswort (*Salicornia herbacea* L.). *Korean Journal of Medicinal Crop Science*, 2002, 10, 93-99.

Jurczuk, M; Moniuszko-Jakoniuk, J; Brzóska, MM. Hepatic and renal concentrations of vitamins E and C in lead- and ethanol-exposed rats. An assessment of their involvement in the mechanisms of peroxidative damage. *Food and Chemical Toxicology*, 2007, 45, 1478-1486.

Koleva, II; van Beek, TA; Linssen, JP; De Groot, A; Evstatieva, LN. Screening of plant extracts for antioxidant activity: a comparative study on three testing methods. *Phytochemical Analysis*, 2002,13, 8-17.

Lee, HJ; Kim, YA; Ahn, JW; Lee, BJ; Moon, SG; Seo, Y. Screening of peroxynitrite and DPPH radical scavenging activities from salt marsh plants. *Korean Journal of Biotechnology and Bioengineering*, 2004, 19, 57-61.

Liu, CM; Ma, JQ; Sun, YZ. Quercetin protects the rat kidney against oxidative stress-mediated DNA damage and apoptosis induced by lead. *Environmental Toxicology and Pharmacology*, 2010, 30, 264-271.

Liu, JN; Yoshida, Y; Wang, MQ; Okai, Y; Yamashita, U. B cell stimulation activity of seaweed extracts. *International Journal of Immunopharmacology*, 1997, 19, 135-142.

Lohr, JW; Willsky, GR; Acara, A. Renal drug metabolism. *Pharmacological Reviews*, 1998, 50, 107-141.

Lu, Z; Hodges, RM; Mota-Urbina, CJ; Gallawa, PL; Chaturvedi, R; DeCianne, DM; Glenn, EP; Hodges, CN. *Salicornia bigelovii* (Chenopodiaceae) seawater irrigated crop with versatile commercial products. In: The Fifth New Crops Symposium. *Atlanta*, GA; 2001.

Madden, EF; Akkerman, M; Fowler, BA. A comparison of 60, 70 and 90 kDa protein expression in normal rat NRK-52E and human HK-2 kidney cell lines following *in vitro* exposure to arsenite and cadmium alone and combination. *Journal of Biochemical and Molecular Toxicology*, 2002, 16, 24-32.

Marnett, LJ. Oxy radicals, lipid peroxidation and DNA damage. *Toxicology*, 2002, 182, 219-222.

Navarro-Moreno, LG; Quintanar-Escorza, MA; González, S; Mondragón, R; Cerbón- Solorzáno, J; Valdés, J; Calderón-Salinas, JV. Effects of lead intoxication on intercellular junctions and biochemical alterations of the renal proximal tubule cells. *Toxicology In Vitro*, 2009, 23, 1298-1304.

Needleman, H. Lead poisoning. *Annual Review of Medicine*, 2004, 55, 209-222.

Nocentini, S; Guggiari, M; Rouillard, D; Surgis, S. Exacerbating effect of vitamin E supplementation on DNA damage induced in cultured human normal fibroblasts by UVA radiation. *Photochemistry and Photobiology*, 2001, 73, 370-377.

Park, JH; Lee, JK; Kim, HS; Chung, ST; Eom, JH; Kim, KA; Chung, SJ; Paik, SY; Oh, HY. Immunomodulatory effect of caffeic acid phenethyl ester in Bal b/c mice. *International Immunopharmacology*, 2004, 4, 429-436.

Pick, E. Microassays for superoxide and hydrogen peroxide production and nitroblue tetrazolium reduction using an enzyme immunoassay microplate reader. *Methods in Enzymology*, 1986, 132, 407-421.

Pulido, MD; Parrish, AR. Metal-induced apoptosis: mechanisms. *Mutation Research.*, 2003, 533, 227-241.

Rice-Evans, CA; Miller, NJ; Paganga, G. Antioxidant properties of phenolic compounds. *Trends in Plant Science*, 1997, 2, 152-159.

Salvesen, GS; Abrams, JM. Caspase activation- stepping on the gas or releasing the brakes? Lessons from humans and flies. *Oncogene*, 2004, 23, 2774-2784.

Seo, Y; Lee, HJ; Kim, YA; Youn, HJ; Lee, BJ. Effects of several salt marsh plants on mouse spleen and thymus cell proliferation using MTT assay. *Ocean Science*, 2005, 40, 209-212.

Seo, Y; Lee, HJ; Park, KE; Kim, YA; Ahn, JW; Yoo, JS; Lee, BJ. Peroxynitrite scavenging constituents from the brown alga *Sargassum thunbergii*. *Biotechnology and Bioengineering*, 2004, 9, 212-216.

Shan, BE; Yoshida, Y; Kuroda, E; Yamashita, U. Immunomodulating activity of seaweed extract on human lymphocytes *in vitro*. *International Journal of Immunopharmacology*, 1999, 21, 59-70.

Tapiero, H; Tew, KD; Ba, GN; Mathe, G. Polyphenols: do they play a role in the prevention of human pathologies? *Biomedicine & Pharmacotherapy*, 2002, 56, 200-207.

Upreti, RK; Kannan, A; Pant, AB. Experimental exposure of arsenic in cultured rat intestinal epithelial cells and cell line: toxicological consequences. *Toxicology In Vitro*, 2007, 21, 32-40.

Ventura, Y; Wuddineh, WA; Myrzabayeva, M; Alikulov, Z; Khozin-Goldberg, I; Shpigel, M; Samocha, TM; Sagi, M. Effect of seawater concentration on the productivity and nutritional value of annual *Salicornia* and perennial *Sarcocornia* halophytes as leafy vegetable crops. *Scientia Horticulturae*, 2011, 128, 189-196.

Woo, M; Hakem, R; Soengas, MS; Duncan, GS; Shahinian, A; Kagi, D; Hakem, A; McCurrach, M; Khoo, W; Kaufman, SA; Senaldi, G; Howard, T; Lowe, SW; Mak, TW. Essential contribution of caspase 3/CPP32 to apoptosis and its associated nuclear changes. *Gene and Development*, 1998, 12, 806-819.

Xiang, JJ; Zhai, Y; Tang, Y; Wang, H ; Liu, B ; Guo, CW. A competitive indirect enzyme-linked immunoassay for lead ion measurement using mAbs against the lead-DTPA complex. *Environmental Pollution*, 2010, 158, 1376-1380.

Xu, J; Ji, LD; Xu, LH. Lead-induced apoptosis in PC 12 cells: Involvement of p53, Bcl-2 family and caspase-3. *Toxicology Letters*, 2006, 166, 160-167.

Index

D

E

I

N

O

P

T

U